T0324642

Molecular Immunity
A Chronology of
60 Years of Discovery

Other World Scientific Title by the Author

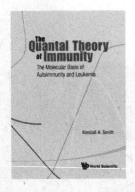

The Quantal Theory of Immunity:
The Molecular Basis of Autoimmunity and Leukemia
ISBN: 978-981-4271-75-2

Molecular Immunity

A Chronology of
60 Years of Discovery

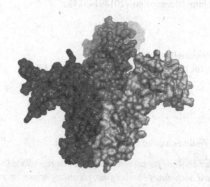

Kendall A. Smith
Cornell University, USA

World Scientific

NEW JERSEY · LONDON · SINGAPORE · BEIJING · SHANGHAI · HONG KONG · TAIPEI · CHENNAI · TOKYO

Published by

World Scientific Publishing Co. Pte. Ltd.

5 Toh Tuck Link, Singapore 596224

USA office: 27 Warren Street, Suite 401-402, Hackensack, NJ 07601

UK office: 57 Shelton Street, Covent Garden, London WC2H 9HE

Library of Congress Cataloging-in-Publication Data
Names: Smith, Kendall A., author.
Title: Molecular immunity : a chronology of 60 years of discovery / Kendall A Smith.
Description: New Jersey : World Scientific, 2018. | Includes bibliographical references and index.
Identifiers: LCCN 2018014814| ISBN 9789813231702 (hardcover : alk. paper) |
    ISBN 981323170X (hardcover : alk. paper)
Subjects: | MESH: Allergy and Immunology--history | Molecular Biology--history |
    Immune System Phenomena | Immunity, Cellular | History, 20th Century | History, 21st Century
Classification: LCC QR181 | NLM QW 511.1 | DDC 616.07/9--dc23
LC record available at https://lccn.loc.gov/2018014814

British Library Cataloguing-in-Publication Data
A catalogue record for this book is available from the British Library.

For any available supplementary material, please visit
http://www.worldscientific.com/worldscibooks/10.1142/10755#t=suppl

Printed in Singapore

For Lynn

Contents

Prologue

This book originated with a request from a postdoctoral fellow that I buy him an expensive textbook of immunology. You see, he was educated in biochemistry, and he could not decipher the new vocabulary and concepts of immunology with which he was confronted daily. I told him that purchasing such an expensive text was a waste of money, in that he probably would not read it, or if he did read it, he would not understand it, and if he did read it and understand it, he would probably forget it by the next day. I went on to say, that the only way to learn about the science of immunology was to read the primary literature. Subsequently, upon thinking over this request, I regained my composure, and took pity on this fellow, because I remembered my own struggle to understand immunology as a young physician when first confronted with this new (to me) science of immunology five decades ago.

I decided that it would be fun, and educational, for the whole lab to review the classic papers of immunology, in the form of a journal club. Thus, instead of our weekly journal club focusing on the latest reports, I assigned each lab member a publication to review each week, starting with Edward Jenner's 1798 monograph, "An Inquiry into the Causes and Effects of Variolae Vaccinae, a Disease Discovered in Some Western Counties of England." As I recall, I started the journal club off by reviewing this marvelous publication, which is essentially a compilation of 23 case reports, in which Jenner describes his very meticulous observations of the effects of inoculations of cowpox material transferred from one person to another, followed in some cases by challenges with virulent Small Pox.

We then went on to Louis Pasteur's reports to l'Academie des Sciences of his first experiments in the late 19th century with his chicken cholera vaccine to his anthrax vaccine, and finally to his rabies vaccine that he administered to humans. Along the way, we observed how reporting science changed over the decades. Pasteur did not include any data in his presentations to the Academy. Rather, he simply told the members of his interpretations of the results. Gradually, as the 20th century began, and scientific journals arose across Europe and the United States, a format evolved that we are familiar with today, comprising an introduction, methods, results and discussion. However, in the first half of the century, most experiments in immunology were performed on whole animals or humans, with observations on the effects of the injections of antigens, much as Jenner had done in the late 18th century. Moreover, most of the data were presented either in the texts of the reports, or in the form of tables, which we all had difficulty deciphering, as to whether the data supported the conclusions of the investigators. There were no figures presented that enables one to rapidly see differences between experimental groups. In addition, statistical evaluations were minimal if used at all.

Fast forward to today, in the early 21st century, the standard format for scientific publications is still the same, with the four main sections, but now each figure is comprised of multiple subfigures, and to conserve space, the subfigures are compressed so that one needs to magnify each one to discern the message. Also, there are as many supplemental figures published online that the reader must consult along with additional methods and figure captions. Compounding the difficulty of the scientific literature is the tremendous complexity of experimental methods and manipulations that are employed. Consequently, to prepare a report to a journal club, so that everyone has a chance to see the critical data, and decide whether the investigators have really proved their hypotheses, can take up to a week of study.

I decided to begin this volume with Sir MacFarlane Burnet's 1957 seminal short hypothesis paper of The Clonal Selection Theory, since this remarkable publication set the stage and posed the questions for the next 60 years of experimentation. In addition, earlier books on the history of immunology ended around 1970, and since the 1960's and 1970's were focused on deciphering the cells responsible for immunity, all the information about the cells and the molecules made and used by the cells to mount and regulate an immune response have not yet been chronicled. The molecular revolution has only occurred since 1980. In addition, most, if not all, of scientific histories are digestions of scientific progress by the writer. It is very seldom that rigorous chronologies are undertaken, especially dealing with who the investigators were, how the experiments were accomplished, and why particular experimental results moved the field forward.

Accordingly, this volume is meant to illuminate the tremendous progress that has been made in the last 60 years in immunology, progress that has led for the first time to the importance of the molecules discovered, as the molecules are the keys to intervene therapeutically in the immune system, either to enhance or to suppress immune reactivity for the benefit of mankind. In addition, this volume is meant as a reference source for the present and next generation of scientists who become fascinated by the immune system, and decide to focus their careers on moving our knowledge forward.

Kendall A. Smith
New York,
August, 2017

1 Twenty Years of Cellular Discovery

The Legacy of Burnet

The term adaptive immunity is usually reserved for the type of immunity that adjusts to respond to an invading microbe, i.e. it adapts. A synonym that has also been used is "acquired" immunity, which is to say that it is different from "innate" or inborn immunity. Adaptive immunity carries with it the connotation of a heightened response to the re-exposure to an antigen experienced previously. This we call immunological memory. It is now recognized and well accepted that lymphocytes are the cells responsible for adaptive immunity, and that the two major types of lymphocytes, B cells and T cells, are both active participants. The phenomenon of immunological memory depends upon specificity of antigen recognition, as well as specificity of the immunological response. As such, adaptive immunity explains why vaccination is effective in preventing infectious diseases, and thus is the essence of immunity, defined as the *exemption* from disease.

When trying to understand any biological phenomenon, it is often helpful to take a scholarly approach and delve into the history of thought and experimental data that have been brought to bear on the problem. In this instance, a logical starting point is the discussion of "The Facts of Immunity" as laid down by Sir Macfarlane Burnet in the third chapter of his seminal monograph of the Abraham Flexner Lectures that he gave at Vanderbilt University in 1958, entitled "The Clonal Selection Theory of Acquired Immunity."[1]

Burnet stated:

"The facts of immunity that I want to summarize are those which seem most relevant to any attempt to look at the immune responses as a part of a general biological picture. They can be listed as follows":

1. *The physical nature of the populations of reactive globulin molecules in a typical antiserum.*
2. *The differences, quantitative and qualitative, between primary and secondary responses.*
3. *The lack of immunological reactivity to body components and the related phenomenon of tolerance.*
4. *The qualitative types of immune response (i.e. cellular vs. humoral).*
5. *Congenital agammaglobulinemia.*
6. *The part played by mesenchymal cells, particularly those of the lymphoid series in immune reactions.*

Of the nature of the reactive globulin molecules, considerable progress had already been made in the first half of the 20th century by the time of Burnet's lectures.[2,3] Now, 50 years later, we know that antibody activity is ascribable to immunoglobulin (Ig) molecules, which are identifiable in the sera of all vertebrates, and in mammals are categorized into five classes or isotypes, designated IgM, IgD, IgG, IgA, and IgE. Also, as a result of the progress made in the second half of the 20th century, we know that Burnet's theory of Clonal Selection is correct; each Ig molecule is the product of a single B cell, which differentiates into an Ig producing plasma cell.[4]

With regard to the differences between primary and secondary immune responses, as summarized by Burnet, *"A particularly clear example is that obtained with staphylococcal toxoid in early work,[5] where the primary response is slow and of low titer, the secondary one rapid and rising almost logarithmically to a higher titer."* We now know that the major difference accounting for the rapidity of the secondary response compared with the primary response, is owing to the proliferative expansion of the antigen-selected clones of cells during the primary response, as initially proposed by Burnet.[1,6] As to the qualitative differences between the primary and secondary responses, we also know that in the process of responding to the initial primary exposure to antigen, the B cells undergo a differentiative process to become "memory" B cells, which has now been explained at the molecular level by genetic changes of recombination of the Ig genes,[7] which accounts for isotype switching, and somatic hypermutation, which accounts for the phenomenon of affinity maturation.[8,9]

Thus, for the past 30 years we have known *what* happens because of the primary antigenic stimulation, but we have only recently begun to unravel the secrets of exactly *how* these differentiative cellular changes take place at the molecular level, and what the molecular signals are that dictate them. Initially, it was assumed that antigen binding to surface Ig furnished all of the molecular signals necessary, in that after antigen selection, B cell proliferation ensues and precedes B cell differentiation. However, we are now aware that there are additional molecular ligand-receptor mechanisms that orchestrate these complicated cellular changes. It follows that it is axiomatic that B cell proliferation and differentiation are not simply pre-programmed changes that are only intrinsic to B cells and not other types of cells.

One crucial aspect of Burnet's view of immunity that still had to be developed concerned the cellular immune response as compared with humoral immunity. By the time that Burnet formulated his theory, Medawar had already shown in 1944 that skin allografts prompt a remarkable rejection reaction with graft-infiltrative round inflammatory cells,[10] and in 1945, Chase had shown that it is possible to transfer cutaneous delayed-type hypersensitivity (DTH) to tuberculin with cells but not sera.[11] Moreover, in 1952 Bruton reported a child with agammaglobulinemia who was unable to produce antibodies, and thus had great difficulty with bacterial infections, but had no difficulty recovering from viral infections.[12]

Burnet first proposed that lymphocytes are the cells responsible for immunity in 1957,[6] and in his more extensive 1959 treatise[1] he summarized the available data indicating that there are at least three types of immune reactions:

1. Classical antibody responses
2. Hay-fever type responses
3. Tuberculin type responses

The first two types he convincingly attributed to Ig molecules. However, the third type was problematic, in that *"Type (3) differs sharply in that there is no evidence that any circulating antibody is produced"*.[1] Burnet went on to discuss that perhaps lymphocytes might be responsible for these cellular reactions, but he was still unsure of the origin of lymphoid cells, and he speculated that perhaps all mesenchymal cells were interchangeable, including lymphocytes, monocytes/macrophages, plasma cells, and even fibroblasts. There seemed to be no controversy that plasma cells were the source of antibody molecules as a result of Fagraeus' 1948 seminal report,[4] but there was a lack of convincing evidence of the interchangeability of each of these cells, especially as to whether lymphocytes could become plasma cells.

Because of the uncertainty of the cellular origins of immune responses, both humoral as well as cellular, Burnet could not furnish experimental support for his Clonal Selection Theory. In his monograph, Burnet comes to the following conclusion:

> *"Only by the use of a pure clone technique of tissue culture, which allows mesenchymal cells to retain full functional activity, would we be likely to find an answer. The clonal selection hypothesis would be completely validated if it could be shown that single cells from a nonimmune animal gave rise to clones, each cell of which under proper physiological conditions contained, or could liberate, antibody-type globulin of a single pattern."*[1]

Of course, now with the advantage of hindsight, we know the answers to the questions posed by Burnet. However, it took another two decades to acquire the experimental data to prove the Clonal Selection **Theory**, to make it the Clonal Selection **Law** of immunology.

Moreover, Burnet was prescient in his prediction that only the capacity to develop pure clones of functional cells would make it possible.

Lymphocytes: The Cellular Basis for Immunity

The initial breakthrough was supplied only one year later in 1960 by Peter Nowell,[13] who made the serendipitous discovery that a plant lectin extracted from the kidney bean, phytohemagglutinin (PHA), had the remarkable capacity to promote a morphological change in small round resting human lymphocytes to one in which the cells resembled immature leukemic blast cells, a process that came to be termed "lymphocyte blastic transformation." Moreover, following this blastic transformation, the cells underwent mitosis and cytokinesis. These findings were truly seminal, because prior to Nowell's discovery, lymphocytes were described in textbooks as terminally differentiated, end-stage cells, incapable of self-renewal. Soon thereafter, in 1962 Gowans demonstrated that small lymphocytes would undergo proliferation *in vivo* after antigenic stimulation and give rise to circulating antibodies.[14] Other reports followed soon thereafter in 1963 and 1964 by Kurt Hirschhorn and Fritz Bach and their co-workers that extended the phenomenon to specific antigen *in vitro*.[15-17] Accordingly, Burnet's prophecy that antigen selected lymphocytes could undergo proliferative clonal expansion became a reality.

Also in 1963, the capacity to visualize and enumerate antibody-forming cells *in vitro* was first reported by future Nobel Laureate (1984) Neils Jerne together with Al Nordin and Claudia Henry.[18] This technique, which came to be called the Jerne Plaque Assay, employed a source of lymphocytes from an animal immunized with Sheep Red Blood Cells (SRBCs), and a source of complement, which was supplied by using guinea pig sera. Thus, splenocytes or lymph node cells from SRBC-immunized rabbits or mice could be mixed with SRBCs and soft agar, and placed in Petri dishes, followed by the addition of complement, which would facilitate antibody-mediated lysis of the SRBCs, thereby forming a clear "plaque" against the homogeneous red background formed by the SRBCs. Each clear plaque could be observed under the microscope to contain a single central lymphoid cell, thus providing the first evidence that individual lymphocytes could give rise to cells that secrete antibody molecules. However, these data did not actually prove Burnet's theory, in that the antibody molecules secreted by single cells still had to be shown to be "monoclonal" or identical individual Ig molecules.

In addition, the thymus had intrigued immunologists for some time, but experiments removing the thymus from animals failed to yield any immunological consequences, so that it was not clear whether this curious lymphoid organ played a role or not in the immune system. Since newborns were immunologically naive, Jacques Miller reasoned in 1962 that the thymus might play a role in lymphocyte development, and thus he conjectured that *"neonatal thymectomy might be associated with some detectable effect on the maturation of immunological faculty."*[19]

Accordingly, Miller devised a method to thymectomize mice within the first three days of life (day 3 thymectomy; d3Tx). He found that such d3Tx mice grew normally during the first month, but thereafter suffered from "runting disease" very similar to Graft vs. Host Disease (GvHD), *"characterized by progressive weight loss, lethargy, ruffled fur, humped posture and diarrhea."*[19] Most mice succumbed before three months of age with lymphocytes invading multiple organs. Within the first six weeks of life, when the mice looked grossly normal, the d3Tx mice were found to have a severe peripheral lymphopenia and undeveloped secondary lymphoid tissues. In addition, these mice were markedly immunocompromized, in that both skin allografts and xenografts went unrejected, and d3Tx mice failed to produce antibody agglutinin activity in response to common bacterial antigens. Accordingly, this was the first inkling that the thymus was important for the development of immunity, and Miller correctly concluded that *"during very early life, the thymus produces the progenitors of immunocompetent cells which mature and migrate to other sites."* However, the cause of the runting disease that led to the premature demise of neonatally thymectomized mice went unexplored and unexplained, but as we shall see, this was the first documentation of the phenomenon of immunodeficiency coexisting with autoimmunity.

In studies examining a secondary immune response of rabbits to the injection of a small molecular hapten coupled to a large protein carrier, Zoltan Ovary and Baruj Benacerraf clearly showed in 1963 that antibodies reactive with the hapten are increased only when the same carrier protein is used for the secondary stimulus as for the first injection.[20] Also, if only the carrier protein is used for the second injection, an anamnestic response to the hapten does not occur. Eventually, this came to be called the "carrier effect," although the basis for this phenomenon went unexplained.

Against this background, the 1965 work of Max Cooper in the chicken was seminal in defining two separate and distinct immune pathways.[21,22] The avian bursa of Fabricius, a lymphocyte-rich outpouching of the gastrointestinal tract much like the appendix, had been discovered serendipitously to be the origin of precursors of antibody-forming cells.[23] Thus, neonatal bursectomy led to the avian equivalent of Bruton's agammaglobulinemia and the incapacity of producing antibody activity in response to immunization.

Accordingly, Cooper subjected newly hatched chickens to bursectomy, thymectomy or both, and then traced their development of secondary lymphoid organs, as well as their capacities to generate antibodies or to reject skin grafts. He found that like in mammals, *"thymus-dependent development is represented morphologically by the small lymphocytes in the circulation, and the white pulp-type development of the tissues... and is basic to the ontogenesis of cellular immunity: graft vs. host responses, delayed hypersensitivity and homograft rejection.* By comparison, *"bursa-dependent development is represented by the larger lymphocytes of the germinal centers and the plasma cells, and functionally by the immunoglobulins."* It was also noted by Cooper and his team that although neonatally thymectomized and irradiated chickens had normal circulating IgM and IgG levels, they only produced about half as much specific antibody responses to some, but not all antigens.[21] Such antigens were subsequently termed Thymus-dependent or T-dependent antigens.

Thus, by 1965 adaptive antigen-specific immunity was established to derive from small lymphocytes that originated in the thymus, subsequently termed T cells, and in the bird in the bursa of Fabricius, subsequently termed B cells. A prolonged search for the mammalian equivalent of the avian bursa was negative, so that the default tissue became the bone marrow, assumed to be the source of antibody-forming mammalian B cells, and fortuitously also beginning with the letter B.

1965 was also the year of the first reports of antigen-nonspecific mitogenic activities produced by alloantigen-stimulated leukocytes. Two groups reported simultaneously that allogeneic mixed lymphocyte cultures produced "blastogenic factors."[24,25] Also, antiviral activity similar to interferon was found in mitogen-stimulated leukocyte culture supernatants.[26] These findings were considered anomalous by most immunologists, because it was unclear how such antigen-nonspecific activities, subsequently termed lymphokines, could participate in antigen-specific adaptive immunity. From this beginning, lymphokines were relegated to a secondary role, thought simply as amplifying antigen-initiated processes that were already initiated and ongoing. No one anticipated that lymphokines might be essential for adaptive immune responses to specific antigen, and crucial for immunoregulation.

Immune Response Genes and Cellular Cooperation

By far, some of the most exciting and intriguing findings of the early 1960s were reports by Baruj Benacerraf and his team of the genetic control of immune responses to synthetic polypeptide antigens in guinea pigs,[27–29] and the confirmation and extension of these findings to inbred mouse strains in the late 1960s by Hugh McDevitt and his group, who demonstrated that the genes in control were linked to those of the major Histocompatability Complex (MHC).[30,31] However, exactly how this large and complex gene locus regulated the immune response remained totally obscure.

One clue was provided by Henry Claman's group, who first showed in 1966 that thymocytes and bone marrow derived cells cooperated in the production of antibodies.[32] They took advantage of a system whereby potential immunocompetent cells are transferred to irradiated hosts, then immunized with SRBCs as antigen. They found that splenocytes were capable of producing foci of Antibody Forming Cells (AFCs), but neither thymocytes or bone marrow cells alone could do so. However, a combination of thymocytes and bone marrow cells were very active. *"The simplest interpretation is that one cell population contains cells capable of making antibody ("effector cells"), but only in the presence of ("auxiliary cells").* However, their data did not allow them to discriminate the former vs. the latter. Conclusive experiments by Jacques Miller and George Mitchell using adult thymectomized, irradiated bone marrow-protected mice showed in 1969 that *"AFC precursors were derived from bone marrow, while the role of thymus cells or of Thoracic Duct Lymphocytes (TDL) is to influence in some way the differentiation of AFC precursors in response to antigen."*[33]

Subsequently, several technical findings advanced the capacity of immunologists to study the immune response. Up until the late 1960s the immune response, of necessity could only be studied *in vivo*, either in animals or humans. In 1967, Robert Mishell and Richard Dutton made possible the analysis of the entire immune response *in vitro* by mixing naïve mouse splenocytes with SRBCs in culture for several days to promote a primary immune response, which they then quantified using a Jerne plaque assay.[34] This facilitated examination of several aspects of the immune response that had heretofore been hidden in the proverbial *in vivo* "black box." In particular, it allowed the direct observation of Burnet's prediction of the proliferative expansion of antigen-reactive clones.[35] In addition, it also led to a dissection of the cells involved, and it was readily shown by Don Mosier in 1967 that macrophages are required for antibody formation to SRBCs by lymphocytes.[36] Thus, in his own words, *"It appears that in the mouse spleen, production of antibody to sheep erythrocytes involves both antigen phagocytosis by macrophages and macrophage lymphocyte interaction, both processes being essential for development of lymphoid cells releasing hemolytic antibody.*

In this regard, in a prescient 1968 report, Emil Unanue and Brigitte Askonas showed convincingly using radiolabeled protein antigen, that *"immunogenicity of live macrophages persisted relatively unaltered for prolonged periods of time* (as long as two weeks) *and appeared to be associated with only a small percentage of antigen held by the cell in a form where it was protected from rapid breakdown and elimination.*[37]

Also in 1968, Theodore Brunner's team developed a radiolabeled [51]Chromium-release assay that enabled the quantification of direct cell-mediated lysis (CML) of target cells, so that one could readily identify and quantify the amounts of lysis mediated by one cell population vs. another.[38] This assay extended the antigen-activation of lymphocyte proliferation to the capacity to monitor effector properties of cell-mediated antigen-specific adaptive immune reactivity *in vitro*, thus greatly facilitating the analysis of DTH, allograft rejection and GvHD, which were the *in vivo* assays of cellular immunity.

Soon thereafter, using living cells rather than fixed or frozen cells, and using fluorescent-labeled antisera reactive with the theta (θ) antigen, in 1969 and 1970 Martin Raff identified θ-positive cells in a subset of murine peripheral secondary lymphoid tissues, and a reciprocal population of cells that were reactive with fluorescent-labeled anti-Ig.[39,40] Simultaneously, Benvenuto Pernis confirmed and extended the expression of surface Ig on a subpopulation of rabbit lymphocytes, and speculated that this surface Ig could be the antigen receptors predicted by Burnet.[41]

Martin Raff immediately tested the role of θ⁺ splenocytes (T cells) in a secondary humoral immune response in hapten-carrier primed mice.[42] The experimental setup included adult mice immunized with the hapten 4-hydroxy-3-iodo-5-nitrophenyl acetic acid (NIP) coupled to the carrier bovine serum albumin (BSA). Splenocytes from these mice were harvested 8–12 weeks after immunization, treated or not with anti-θ and guinea pig sera as a source of complement, and then injected into syngeneic recipients previously irradiated with 600 rad. The following day the recipients were immunized with NIP-BSA, and then tested for circulating antibodies 10 days later. The results indicated that the T cells are "helper" cells, responding to the carrier determinants on BSA, whereas non-θ⁺ cells are the cells responsible for producing antibodies reactive with the hapten NIP.

These findings were also confirmed and extended to the total *in vitro* immunization system by Anneliese Schimpl and Eberhard Wecker.[43]

Despite these new findings, the role of thymocytes and thymic-dependent cells in immunity was still obscure, leading Jerne just one year later in 1971 to propose that *"in the primary lymphoid organs, e.g. in the thymus, the proliferation of lymphocytes... leads to the selection of mutant cells expressing v-genes that have been modified by spontaneous random mutation."*[44] He was partially correct about somatic mutation as being responsible for the creation of antibody-antigen binding diversity, but totally wrong about thymocytes as precursors of AFCs.

T Cell "Help" for B Cells

Also in 1971, Jacques Miller and Jonathan Sprent were uniquely poised to perform adoptive transfer experiments to determine whether primed T cells and primed AFC precursors both possessed "memory," and cooperated to produce a secondary immune response. To ensure complete depletion of thymus-derived cells, these investigators employed a system of transferring thoracic duct lymphocytes from antigen-primed mice to irradiated recipients. To test whether primed T cells were required, the thoracic duct cells were treated with anti-H2 sera that they had shown would eliminate virtually 100% of the T cells. Anti-θ sera were also used, but were found to only partially deplete T cells. These cells were then adoptively transferred to neonatal thymectomized mice: the antibody responses were lower by 1 $\log_{10}$ when T-depleted thoracic duct lymphocytes were transferred. Moreover, primed B cells were also required in these adoptive transfer experiments, leading to the conclusion that *"memory is a property that can be linked to both B cells and T cells."*[45]

Given these findings, a series of 1971 experiments reported by Avrion Mitchison were seminal in a field that was to become obsessed with the question as to the molecular mechanism(s) of how T cells recognize antigens when they "help" antibody production, as well as the molecular mechanism(s) of the "help." Mitchison's experiments on the secondary immune responses of mice to immunization with hapten-carrier conjugates led him to conclude that the helper T cells recognize carrier determinants and the AFC precursors recognize either the hapten or other carrier determinants.[46] He speculated that there was *"the possibility of an antigen bridge linking the receptor (presumably a normal Ig molecule) on the AFC precursor with another receptor (IgX) on the thymus derived cell."* This concept came to be termed "linked recognition," and led to a familiar schematic diagram of a B cell-antigen-T cell linkage presented at virtually all scientific meetings thereafter. Another term subsequently used for this function became known as "cognate recognition," which emphasized the physical interaction between the AFC and the T cell, as well as the presumed molecular similarity between the B cell and T cell antigen recognition molecules.

Thus, the stage was set for the question that became the "holy grail" of immunology for the next decade, the nature of the T cell antigen receptor, which became abbreviated to simply the T cell receptor (TCR, as if T cells had no other receptors). Many of the most accomplished and prestigious research groups were attracted to the quest. Moreover, the focus of many immunologists also became the question as to how T cell "recognition" of antigen led to the apparent required T cell "help" provided to B cells that promoted antibody formation, as well as the molecular mechanism(s) responsible. The solutions to these questions consequently became intertwined.

Macrophages "Help" B Cells Too

Confounding these issues was the growing awareness that macrophages also seemed to play a role in the "help" that B cells required. It had already been shown by Joost Oppenheim in 1968 that T cells needed "help" from macrophages to proliferate in response to stimulation by specific antigens and low concentrations of non-specific mitogens, such as PHA.[47] Accordingly, it was a logical next step to ask the question as to whether a soluble macrophage product might serve to replace the necessity of actual macrophages themselves. In 1970, Fritz Bach and his co-workers presented evidence that media conditioned by *"an adherent cell population-enriched in macrophages"* could substitute for macrophages allowing purified lymphocytes to proliferate in response to soluble protein antigens or to allogeneic lymphocytes. They speculated that the macrophages produced a factor that they termed *"conditioned medium reconstituting factor-CMRF"* that potentiated *in vitro* lymphocyte reactivity.[48] The presumption was that the CMRF was produced by macrophages but worked its effects on the lymphocytes, amplifying their reaction to specific antigens.

Simultaneously, Richard Dutton and his group reported very similar results analyzing the generation of AFCs using their "Mishell-Dutton assay." Thus, following up Mosier's 1967 observation that macrophages are required for the generation of AFCs reactive with SRBCs *in vitro,* they found that conditioned media from 24-hour cultures of glass-adherent cells, incubated with or without SRBCs, could substitute for macrophages in permitting the nonattached lymphocytes to generate AFCs.[49,50] One other noteworthy aspect about the Mishell-Dutton *in vitro* AFC assay was its dependence on "optimal batches" of Fetal Calf Sera (FCS) to observe any AFCs at all.

Soon thereafter, in 1972 Igal Gerry working with Richard Gershon and Byron Waksman reported a series of experiments that showed that glass adherent cells released a mitogenic activity that enhanced the proliferation of murine thymocytes as well as purified peripheral T cells when stimulated by PHA.[51,52] They called this activity lymphocyte activating factor (LAF), and showed that its activity increased when the adherent cells are stimulated with bacterial lipopolysaccharide (LPS). As to its mechanism of action, it was speculated that LAF was simply a mitogen itself, like PHA. Alternatively, they wondered whether LAF supplied some trace nutrients necessary for cellular proliferation, thereby simply facilitating a proliferative process that was already initiated by the PHA. They referenced the earlier work on mitogenic activities found in leukocyte and macrophage conditioned media, but there was no way to ascertain whether the activities were identical or not.

Following up their findings of the requirement for T cells in the Mishell-Dutton assay, Schimpl and Wecker noted that allogeneic but not syngeneic thymocytes could substitute for θ^+ splenocytes.

They speculated that the strong alloantigenic stimulation of the thymocytes might have prompted them to produce a "potentiating factor," similar to the leukocyte-derived blastogenic factor described in 1965,[24,25] and the macrophage-derived activities described independently by Bach and by Dutton, except now they were specifically looking for activities derived from T cells, not macrophages or just leukocytes. Using the Mishell-Dutton assay system for the *in vitro* generation of AFCs, they related new evidence that there might actually be two activities produced by alloantigen-stimulated T cells; (1) a T cell expanding factor (TEF), similar to the Blastogenic Factor described previously, and that acted best if added early to the cultures, but also (2) a T cell replacing factor (TRF), which acted best if added late to the cultures.[53] They further speculated that the TRF would act on B cells, facilitating their differentiation to AFCs, and in the Mitchison linked-recognition model, the soluble TRF would only be at work over a very short range, like a neurotransmitter, and would only be capable of "helping" the B cell linked to a T cell via an antigen bridge between their respective antigen receptors. Thus, they covered all bases. Thus, by 1972 it seemed clear that for an antibody response to a T-dependent antigen, three distinct cells were required, B cells, T cells and macrophages, and that soluble activities were produced by both macrophages and T cells that could replace the cells themselves.

T Cell Suppression and Idiotypic "Networks"

Two additional concepts were introduced at about this time that had tremendous influence on immunological thinking as well as experiments for the next decade. Richard Gershon reported in 1970 that there were "suppressor T cells," in addition to "helper T cells," and that these cells might be responsible for immunological tolerance.[54–56] Moreover, these cells were antigen-specific and could be induced by antigenic stimulation, so that the outcome of antigenic stimulation, immunological activation or tolerance depended upon a balance between T cell help vs. T cell suppression. However, many of Gershon's experiments were quite complex, involving thymectomized, lethally irradiated, bone marrow reconstituted mice that were subsequently immunized with large doses of SRBCs. Moreover, in many of his experiments, cells were adoptively transferred between serial recipients, which were also irradiated and reconstituted with various cell populations. Even though the experiments were complicated, his work gained credence because it was preformed *in vivo*. However, the mechanisms whereby these suppressor T cells functioned were obscured by the proverbial *in vivo* black box. Gershon speculated that perhaps they secreted a suppressive antigen-binding molecule, which he termed IgY to distinguish it from Mitchison's putative secreted helper factor, IgX. It is noteworthy that the immunological community was very receptive to Gershon's concepts, because they promised ways to manipulate the immune response therapeutically, either to enhance or suppress it. Therefore, there was something in it for everyone.

Neils Jerne's "Idiotypic Network Hypothesis" introduced in 1974, is the other, very highly influential concept that dominated the 1970s.[57,58] To account for experimental observations that the antigen-binding v-region of antibody molecules, which he termed a *paratope*, could itself serve as an antigen or a unique epitope that could be recognized by other B cells and give rise to antibodies reactive with them, the terminology of *idiotopes* and *idiotypes* was introduced. Jerne proposed that the vastly diverse population of antibody molecules in a normal individual represents a vast collection of antigens (idiotopes), because of the unique amino acid sequences of each v-region. Thus, in Jerne's words, *"antibody molecules can be recognized as well as recognize."* Jerne hypothesized that prior to the introduction of an external antigen, the concentration of each idiotope was so low that the system displayed an "eigen" behavior, a mathematical-physics term that is translated from German as "self" behavior. Thus, Jerne proposed that resulting from an eigen paratope-idiotope interaction, the system achieves a dynamic steady state, as its elements interact between themselves. However, with the introduction of a foreign epitope, the B cells recognizing it would be stimulated to proliferate, thereby increasing the proportion of epitope-reactive cells, which would then differentiate into high epitope-reactive antibody producing plasma cells, flooding the system with their idiotopes. The net effect would be to markedly increase the concentration of the E-reactive idiotopes, which would exceed the activation threshold of many more reactive B cells, leading to the production of many anti-idiotopes. Ultimately, Jerne envisioned that the growing network stimulated by the original epitope would feed back to neutralize the response to the original foreign epitope.

MHC Restriction

One aspect of the immune system not considered by Jerne was the nature of the molecules that T cells used to recognize antigens. Like most others at the time, Jerne assumed that the TCR would also be found to be an Ig-like molecule, so that he envisioned T cells and B cells to be interchangeable from the standpoint of their antigen recognition molecules. Moreover, there was no place in the Network Hypothesis for Ir-genes as regulators of immune recognition. According to Jerne, *"Benacerraf and McDevitt regarded inescapable the conclusion that there exists a class of molecules encoded by Ir-genes, which are re-sponsible for recognition of specificity at the T cell level, and that these molecules are not immunoglobulins."*[57]

In attempts to understand Ir-gene function, and shed light on the nature of Ir gene products, David Katz and Baruj Benacerraf took a genetic approach in 1973 to examine the question as to whether B cells and T cells needed to be histocompatible for the generation of AFCs in response to hapten (DNP)/carrier (keyhole limpet hemocyanin, KLH) conjugates.[59] They used F1 hosts (AxB strains) as recipients of hapten-primed B cells from one parent (e.g. A strain) and carrier-primed T cells from the other parent (B strain), and found that only histocompatible (syngeneic) combinations would cooperate to gen-erate AFCs. They then also performed similar experiments *in vitro* with similar results. They speculated that the B cells might express an MHC-encoded "acceptor" molecule that interacted with a similar MHC-derived molecule either secreted by, or expressed on, the surface of the T cell.

This report was followed soon afterwards in 1973 by a similar report by Allen Rosenthal and Ethan Shevach who studied the histocompatibility requirements of macrophages and T cells for antigen-induced T cell proliferation.[60] Using guinea pig cells, they found that *"efficient interaction of macrophage associated antigen and immunospecific T lymphocytes as measured by antigen-induced lymphocyte proliferation, only occurs when the macrophages and T cells are histocompatible (syngeneic). It is likely that this interaction is mediated by histocompatibility antigens themselves, or by the products of genes closely linked to the MHC."*

Accordingly, these reports established that Ir genes linked to the MHC complex somehow were very important for T cell antigen recognition. Whether it was necessary that MHC encoded molecules were expressed by all the cells for a productive interaction to occur remained to be determined. However, it was tantalizing to think that the MHC region coded for the elusive TCR. In this regard, it is important to understand that the genetic experiments done at the time indicated that the helper effects on the generation of AFCs and on antigen-specific T cell proliferation did not map to the traditional serologically-defined MHC-encoded molecules. Instead, they mapped between the serological determinants in what was termed the MLC-derived locus, that later became the I-region, or the Ir region, for immune response region.

In the face of these findings, the 1974 reports by Rolf Zinkernagel and Peter Doherty, who studied the histocompatibility requirements for cytolytic T cells to recognize and kill lymphocyte choriomeningitis virus (LCMV)-infected cells, were particularly informative.[61,62] These investigators found that Cytolytic T lymphocytes (CTL) could only kill virus-infected target cells if they shared MHC loci, and that the MHC-encoded determinants mapped to the regions defined serogically, not the I-region. To explain their results, they proposed that T cells expressed two TCRs, one comprising and is interactive with self MHC-encoded determinants on the target cell, and another reactive with virus-specified determinants (nonself), vs. the one TCR hypothesis, in which only one TCR reacted with either a virus-modified MHC-encoded molecule or a combination of virus + MHC-encoded molecules, the so-called "altered self" hypothesis. In follow-up studies two years later, of MHC restriction of virus-specific cytotoxicity across the *H-2* barrier, Zinkernagel concluded:

> *"The results are compatible with the idea that T cells are specific for "altered self" or "altered alloantigen," i.e. a complex of cell surface marker and viral antigen. Alternatively, explained with a dual recognition model, T cells may possess two independently, clonally expressed receptors, a self-recognizer which is expressed for one of the syngeneic or tolerated allogeneic K or D "self" markers, and an immunologically specific receptor for viral antigen."*[63]

Antigen-Specific Helper and Suppressor Factors

Given these findings against the background of the reports of both macrophage-derived and T cell-derived "factors" found in leukocyte conditioned media, investigators began searching for soluble factors, of both "helper" and "suppressor" varieties, and both antigen-specific as well as antigen nonspecific varieties. In 1974, Michael Taussig and Alan Monro were among the first investigators to identify an antigen-specific T cell-derived "helper" factor that appeared to comprise in part by MHC-encoded molecules.[64] They produced their factor as follows: *"T cells (from mice) primed in vivo by specific antigen, were incubated together with antigen in vitro for 6–8 hours. The cells were then removed by centrifugation and the supernatant, containing the T cell factor, (was) transferred together with bone marrow cells and antigen into lethally irradiated, syngeneic recipients. After 14 days, the direct plaque-forming cell (PFC) response to the antigen in the spleens of the recipients was measured and compared to controls receiving B cells and antigen but no factor, or B cells with T cells and antigen."* In attempts to characterize the helper factor, they found that the activity was removed with an immunoadsorbant column prepared with anti-H-2^d sera, but not anti-H-2^k or anti-Ig. Based on their findings, they suggested that *"the T cell factor is the soluble expression of the T cell receptor."*

Also at this time, Marc Feldmann used combined *in vivo* and *in vitro* methods to generate supernatants for study.[65,66] First, "activated T cells" were generated by lethally irradiating mice (800–900 rad), followed by injection intravenously (IV) with 10^8 syngeneic thymocytes, and intraperitoneally (IP) with antigens emulsified in Freund's complete adjuvant. Then 6–7 days later, splenocytes from these mice containing the "activated T cells" were cultured together with antigen in the upper chamber of double-chambered Marbrook-Diener flasks. The fluid in the lower compartment was harvested after 40–48 hours and termed "T cell supernatant." Feldmann described three different kinds of activities in these supernatants. There was an "antigen-specific helper activity" that enhanced the generation of AFCs. In the same supernatants, there was both an "antigen-nonspecific helper activity" as well as an "antigen-specific suppressor activity." To make things even more complicated, it was found that macrophages could abrogate the suppressor activities. Moreover, both antigen-specific helper and suppressor activities were absorbed by Sepharose beads conjugated with anti-mouse Ig, anti-κ-chain or anti-μ-chain sera. Thus, in contrast to Taussig and Monro, Feldmann speculated that his T cell-derived factors, both helper and suppressor, contained an Ig molecule that he termed IgT. Moreover, it was claimed that suppression by "specific factor," which he attributed to IgT-antigen complexes, depended upon direct interaction with lymphocytes.

Tomio Tada's laboratory used a somewhat different system to examine the molecular mechanisms responsible for the suppression of anti-hapten specific antibody responses by T cells primed with high doses of carrier proteins.[67] Both thymocytes and splenocytes from carrier-primed mice were isolated and sonicated. Cellular debris was removed by centrifugation and the cell-free supernatants were tested for their effects on the generation of AFCs by their IV administration to naïve mice immunized concomitantly with hapten-carrier conjugate together with pertussis vaccine as adjuvant. The extracts were found to contain a suppressive factor that depressed the capacity of the immunized mice to generate IgG antibody responses to the hapten. The activity was antigen-specific for the carrier protein used to produce the factor. Like the activity described by Taussig and Monro, immunoadsorbant columns prepared with antisera raised against the K-end of the MHC complex of the donor strain, but not by anti-Ig removed the activity. Also, immunoadsorbants made with the carrier protein antigen also removed the suppressive activity.

All these reports were focused on antigen-specific factors because they hoped that these elusive factors could lead to the molecular nature of the T cell antigen receptor. However, because each laboratory used different methods to produce and assay for their factor activities, the field was chaotic.

T Cell Subsets

Inbred mouse strains became a very important resource for investigating genetic contributions to immunological reactions. In particular, Lloyd Old's group introduced the concept of the identification of subsets of T cells with their description of the *Ly* gene loci that specified discrete alloantigens expressed by functionally distinct T cells in the late 1960s.[68,69] It is noteworthy that the use of congenic mouse strains to produce alloantisera created unique reagents available only to a few investigators who had access to the special congenic mouse strains. Also, large numbers of mice were required to produce only small volumes of precious antisera that could be used only for critical experiments. Edward Boyse investigated congenic mouse strains that differed at only one genetic locus and raised antisera by immunizing across reciprocal congenic mouse strains. The *Ly-1* and *Ly-2* gene loci, on chromosomes 19 and 6, were found to specify alloantigens expressed exclusively and invariably on mouse T cells. Moreover, each locus was found to have alternative alleles that determined the T cell surface antigens Ly-1.1 and Ly-1.2, and Ly-2.1 and Ly-2.2, respectively. Pawel Kisielow, working with Boyse, first showed in 1975 that subsets of peripheral T cells express distinct alleles of Ly surface determinants.[70] Previous reports established that there appeared to be at least two functional T cell subsets, one that proliferated to a large extent when stimulated by alloantigens in an MLC, and another that possessed most of the cytolytic activity.[71] Kisielow found that splenocytes could be distinguished, in that ~ 2/3 were Ly-1+ and possessed most of the proliferative capacity, whereas ~ 1/3 were Ly-2+ and possessed most of the cytolytic capacity.

These findings were confirmed and extended by Harvey Cantor, also working with Boyse,[72,73] who also reported in 1975 that there were actually three subclasses of peripheral T cells, in that ~ 50% expressed all three Ly antigens, 1, 2, and 3. These cells were thought to function as precursors of the other two distinct subclasses. They also showed that during the MLC, the function of the Ly-1+ population to amplify the cytolytic function of the Ly-2/3+ population, depended on Ia+ stimulator cells. In a subsequent report, the T cell subclasses were studied after immunization with SRBCs. Cells of the Ly-1+ subclass were found to provide "helper activity" for the generation of both primary and secondary AFCs. By comparison, cells of the Ly-23+ subclass were found to suppress the generation of AFCs. Because cytolytic cells could not be further separated or distinguished from suppressor cells, the T cell cytotoxic/suppressor (Tc/s) terminology was introduced to immunology for the first time in 1976.[74]

Also in 1976, McDevitt's group produced evidence indicating that a new region within the I-region of the MHC locus, which they termed I-J, coded for surface determinants found only on suppressor T cells.[75] These findings depended on antisera produced by congenic mouse strains that differed only in very restricted areas within the I region of the MHC locus. Simultaneously, Tada's group using similar strains and antisera, reported data indicating that their carrier-specific suppressor factors contained determinants encoded by the I-J subregion.[76] All these data resulted in provocative evidence that genes within the MHC locus encoded molecules, some surface and some apparently secreted, that were very important for T cell regulation of immune responsiveness. Some of the encoded molecules were expressed by macrophages and B cells, while others were expressed by T cells. However, the molecular nature of these determinants and activities remained obscure.

Because each of the investigators used different methods to generate and test their various factor activities, the field was definitely complicated, especially as each investigator claimed different functional attributes for their factor activities. Moreover, there was a striking lack of attempts to purify the molecules responsible for the various activities, so that molecular characterizations beyond assaying for reactivity with various antisera were nonexistent. The difficulties inherent in the biochemical techniques available for protein separation and purification were part of the reasons that biochemical characterizations of the various activities had not been performed. At the time, the only available techniques were molecular sieves that separated proteins based upon their molecular sizes or charges. Polyacrylamide gel separation had not yet been described, and high pressure liquid chromatography (HPLC) also was not yet available. However, another, just as important impediment was the lack of rapid quantitative assays available for the activities, with many investigators dependent only on *in vivo* assays, which made the determination of activities in many fractions from biochemical separative columns virtually impossible.

Ia Molecules

In 1978, Baruj Benacerraf published an "Opinion" article[77] that galvanized and focused investigators perplexed by Ir genes, Ia antigens and the nature of T cell antigen recognition. First, he reiterated the characteristics of Ir genes in the I-regions of the MHC of mammals, and proposed presciently the hypothesis that perhaps the Ia molecules formed an immunogenic complex together with peptide epitopes capable of stimulating T cells. He summarized research indicating that T cells recognize epitopes comprising of short specific chains of 3–4 amino acids, whereas antibodies often recognized epitopes formed by the tertiary structures of native proteins. Also, he stressed the importance of macrophage processing and presentation for T-dependent immune responses, a phenomenon that had been recognized and studied for more than a decade.[37] He intentionally stated that his theory did not define the nature of the T cell antigen receptors, nor the hypothesis that there could be more than one receptor. In addition, he was careful to state that his hypothesis was compatible with the Zinkernagel-Doherty phenomenon, where the K and D region encoded molecules were postulated to interact with viral antigens in a manner similar to Ia molecule-peptide interaction.

He also specifically stated that his hypothesis was not concerned with antigen-specific helper and suppressor factors bearing I region-controlled determinants. In addition, he stressed that according to his hypothesis, macrophage Ia molecules could bind macrophage-processed fragments of autologous proteins, as well as foreign proteins, and that specific unresponsiveness to autologous antigens could not depend upon the absence of Ia-self peptide interactions, but rather must depend on specific unresponsiveness at the T cell level by either an active or passive mechanism.

Thus, Benacerraf crystalized his 20 years of work on the genetic control of the T cell immune response. The Ir gene control specified the curious nature of the antigens recognized by T cells, which differed markedly from the nature of antigens recognized by B cells and antibodies. Even so, the nature of MHC encoded molecules, the peptide-MHC interaction and the TCR remained elusive, including the one receptor vs. two receptor hypotheses.

The period 20 years following Burnets proposal of his Clonal Selection Theory were taken up with the elucidation of the arm of the immune system that was totally obscure in his time, that is the cellular arm, which we now know as the T cell immune response. Its discovery and comparisons and contrasts with the humoral or B cell immune response led to the uncovering of many surprising phenomena, including that T cells "helped" B cells proliferate and differentiate into antibody forming cells, and "suppressed" antibody formation. Moreover, T cells themselves could proliferate and differentiate into "effector" cells capable of killing target cells that they recognized as foreign. Even more mysterious and surprising was the fact that T cells "recognized" foreignness differently than did B cells and antibodies, and even more surprising, both the T cell and B cell immune responses depended upon the genetic constitution of the host, somehow linked to the large gene locus that encodes histocompatibility. In addition, not only were there two distinct kinds of lymphocytes; T cell subsets were recognized for the first time. All these findings occurred as the science of immunology made the transition from studies of whole animals and humans to the study of cells in cultures. This transition led to the discovery of additional lymphocyte products that were not antibodies, which came to be known as lymphokines or cytokines. However, exactly what these newly discovered molecules are, and how they figured into the immune system remained obscure. Thus, by 1980, the burning questions of immunology focused on these issues, and how could one reduce the complexity further, as well as how could one reduce the science from cell populations to individual cells, and finally to molecules.

References

1. Burnet FM. (1959). *The Clonal Selection Theory of Acquired Immunity.* Cambridge: Cambridge University Press.
2. Edelman GM. (1959). Dissociation of gamma globulin. *J Am Chem Soc* **81**:3155–3170.
3. Porter RR. (1959). The hydrolisis of rabbit gamma globulin and antibodies with crystalline papain. *Biochem J* **73**:119–138.
4. Fagraeus A. (1948). The plasma cellular reaction and its relation to the formation of antibodies *in vitro. J Immunol* **58**:1–13.
5. Burnet F. (1940). *Production of Antibodies.* Melbourne: Monographs of the Walter and Eliza Hall Institute.
6. Burnet FM. (1957). A modification of Jerne's theory of antibody production using the concept of clonal selection. *Aust J Sci* **20**:67–77.
7. Hozumi N and Tonegawa S. (1976). Evidence for somatic rearrangement of immunoglobulin genes coding for variable and constant regions. *Proc Natl Acad Sci USA* **73**:3628–3632.
8. Bernard O, Hozumi N and Tonegawa S. (1978). Sequences of mouse immunoglobulin light cain genes before and after somatic changes. *Cell* **15**:1133–1139.
9. Seidman J, Edgell M and Leder P. (1978). Immunoglobulin light chain structural gene sequences cloned in a bacterial plasmid. *Nature* **271**:582–586.
10. Medawar P. (1944). The behavior and fate of skin autografts and skin homografts in rabbits. *J Anat* **78**:176–199.
11. Chase M. (1945). The cellular transfer of cutaneous hypersensitivity to tuberculin. *Proc Soc Exp Biol Med* **59**:134–135.

12. Bruton O. (1952). Agammaglobulinemia. *Pediatrics* **9**:722–728.
13. Nowell PC. (1960). Phytohemagglutinin: An initiator of mitosis in cultures of normal human leukocytes. *Cancer Res* **20**:462–468.
14. Gowans J, McGregor D, Cowan D and Ford C. (1962). Initiation of immune responses by small lymphocytes. *Nature* **196**:651–655.
15. Hirschhorn K, Bach F, Kolodny R, *et al.* (1963). Immune response and mitosis of human peripheral blood lymphocytes *in vitro*. *Science* **142**:1185–1187.
16. Bach F and Hirschhorn K. (1964). Lymphocyte interaction: A potential histocompatibility test *in vitro*. *Science* **143**:813–814.
17. Bain B and Lowenstein L. (1964). Genetic studies on the mixed leukocyte reaction. *Science* **145**:1315–1316.
18. Jerne NK and Nordin AA. (1963). Antibody formation in agar by single anibody-producing cells. *Science* **140**:405.
19. Miller J. (1962). Effect of neonatal thymectomy on the immunological responsiveness of the mouse. *Proc Roy Soc London-B* **156**:415–428.
20. Ovary Z and Benacerraf B. (1963). Immunological specificity of the secondary response with dinitrophenylated proteins. *Proc Soc Exp Biol Med* **114**:72–76.
21. Cooper M, Peterson R and Good R. (1965). Delineation of the thymic and bursal lymphoid systems in the chicken. *Nature* **205**:143–146.
22. Cooper M, Peterson R, South M and Good R. (1966). The functions of the thymus system and the bursa system in the chicken. *J Exp Med* **123**:75–102.
23. Glick B, Chang T and Jaap R. (1956). The bursa of Fabricius and antibody production. *Poultry Sci.* **35**:224.
24. Kasakura S and Lowenstein L. (1965). A factor stimulating DNA synthesis derived from the medium of leukocyte cultures. *Nature* **208**: 794–795.
25. Gordon J and MacLean LD. (1965). A lymphocyte-stimulating factor produced *in vitro*. *Nature* **208**:795–796.
26. Wheelock E. (1965). Interferon-like virus inhibitor induced in human leukocytes by phytohemagglutinin. *Science* **149**:310–311.
27. Kantor FS, Ojeda A and Benacerraf B. (1963). Studies on artificial antigens I. Antigenicity of DNP-polylysine and DNP copolymer of lysine and glutamic acid in guinea pigs. *J Exp Med* **117**:55–64.
28. Levine B, Ojeda M and Benacerraf B. (1963). Studies on artificial antigens III. The genetic control of the immune response to hapten poly-L-lysine conjugates in guinea pigs. *J Exp Med* **118**:953–957.

29. Green I, Paul WE and Benacerraf B. (1966). The behavior of hapten-poly-L-lysine conjugates as complete antigens in genetic responder and as haptens in non-responder guinea pigs. *J Exp Med* **123**:859–879.
30. McDevitt HO and Tyan ML. (1968). Genetic control of the antibody response in inbred mice: Transfer of response by spleen cells and linkage to the major histocompatability (H2) locus. *J Exp Med* **128**:1–11.
31. McDevitt HO and Chinitz A. (1969). Genetic control of the antibody response: Relationship between immune response and histocompatability (H-2) type. *Science* **163**:273–279.
32. Claman HC, Chaperon EA and Triplett PF. (1966). Thymus marrow cell combination. Synergism in antibody production. *Proc Soc Exp Biol Med* **122**:1167–1178.
33. Miller J and Mitchell G. (1969). Cell to cell interaction in the immune response. *Transpl Proc* **1**:535–538.
34. Mishell R and Dutton R. (1967). Immunization of dissociated spleen cell cultures from normal mice. *J Exp Med* **126**:423–442.
35. Dutton RW and Mishell RI. (1967). Cell populations and cell proliferation in the *in vitro* response of normal mouse spleen to heterologous erythrocytes. Analysis by the hot pulse technique. *J Exp Med* **126**:443–432.
36. Mosier D. (1967). A requirement for two cell types for antibody formation *in vitro*. *Science* **158**:1573–1575.
37. Unanue E and Askonas BA. (1968). Persistence of immunogenicity of antigen after uptake by macrophages. *J Exp Med* **127**.
38. Brunner KT, Mauel J, Cerottini J-C and Chapius B. (1968). Quantitative assay of the lytic action of lymphoid cells on 51-Cr labelled allogeneic target cells *in vitro*. Inhibition by isoantibody and drugs. *Immunol.* **14**:181–190.
39. Raff M. (1969). Theta isoantigen as a marker of thymus-derived lymphocytes in mice. *Nature* **224**:378–379.
40. Raff M, Sternberg M and Taylor RB. (1970). Immunoglobulin determinants on the surface of mouse lymphoid cells. *Nature* **225**:553–555.
41. Pernis B, Forni L and Amante L. (1970). Immunoglobulin spots on the surface of rabbit lymphocytes. *J Exp Med* **132**:1001–1018.
42. Raff M. (1970). Role of thymus-derived lymphocytes in the secondary humoral immune response in mice. *Nature* **226**:1257–1258.
43. Schimple A and Wecker E. (1970). Inhibition of *in vitro* immune response by treatment of spleen cell suspensions with anti-theta serum. *Nature* **226**:1258–1259.

44. Jerne NK. (1971). The somatic generation of immune recognition. *Eur J Immunol* **1**:1–9.

45. Miller J and Sprent J. (1971). Cell-to-cell interaction in the immune response VI. Contribution of thymus-derived cells and antibody-forming cell precursors to immunological memory. *J Exp Med* **134**:66–82.

46. Mitchison N. (1971). The carrier effect in the secondary response to hapten-protein conjugates. II Cellular cooperation. *Euro J Immunol* **1**:18–27.

47. Oppenheim J, Leventhal B and Hersh E. (1968). The transformation of column-purified lymphocytes with nonspecific and specific antigenic stimuli. *J Immunol* **101**:262–270.

48. Bach F, Alter B, Solliday S, *et al.* (1970). Lymphocyte reactivity *in vitro* II. Soluble reconstituting factor permitting response of purified lymphocytes. *Cell Immunol* **1**:219–227.

49. Dutton RW, McCarthy MM, *et al.* (1970). Cell components in the immune response. IV. Relationships and possible interactions. *Cell Immunol* **1**:196–206.

50. Hoffman M and Dutton R. (1971). Immune response restoration with macrophage culture supernatants. *Science* **172**:1047–1048.

51. Gery I, Gershon RK and Waksman B. (1972). Potentiation of the T-lymphocyte response to mitogens I. The responding cell. *J Exp Med* **136**:128–142.

52. Gery I and Waksman BH. (1972). Potentiation of the T-lymphocyte response to mitogens: The cellular source of potentiating mediators. *J Exp Med* **136**:143–155.

53. Schimpl A and Wecker E. (1972). Replacement of T cell function by a T cell product. *Nature New Biol* **237**:15–17.

54. Gershon R and Kondo K. (1970). Cell interactions in the induction of tolerance: The role of thymic lymphocytes. *Immunology* **18**:723–737.

55. Gershon R and Kondo K. (1971). Infectious immunolgical tolerance. *Immunology* **21**:903–914.

56. Gershon R, Cohen P, Hencin R and Liebhaber S. (1972). Suppressor T cells. *J Immunol* **108**:586–590.

57. Jerne N. (1974). Towards a network theory of the immune system. *Annales d'Immunologie (Inst. Pasteur)* **125C**:373–389.

58. Jerne N. (1976). The immune system: a web of v-domains. *The Harvey Lectures* **70**:93–110.

59. Katz D, Hamaoka T and Benacerraf B. (1973). Cell interactions between histoincompatible T and B lymphocytes II. Failure of physiologic cooperative interactions between T and B lymphocytes from allogeneic

donor strains in humoral response to hapten-protein conjugates. *J Exp Med* **137**:1405–1418.

60. Rosenthal A and Shevach E. (1973). Function of macrophages in antigen recognition by guinea pig T lymphocytes. I. Requirement for histocompatible macrophages and lymphocytes. *J Exp Med* **138**:1194–1212.

61. Zinkernagel R and Doherty P. (1974). Restriction of *in vitro* T cell-mediated cytotoxicity in lymphocytic choriomeningitis within a syngeneic or semiallogeneic system. *Nature* **248**:701–702.

62. Zinkernagel RM and Doherty PC. (1974). Immunological surveillance against altered self components by sensitized T lymphocytes in lymphocytic choriomeningitis. *Nature* **251**:547–548.

63. Zinkernagel R. (1976). H-2 restriction of virus-specific cytotoxicity accross the H-2 barrier: Separate effector T cell specificities are associated with self-H-2 and with tolerated allogeneic H-2 in chimeras. *J Exp Med* **144**:933–945.

64. Taussig M and Monro A. (1974). Removal of specific cooperative T cell factor by anti-H-2 but not by anti-Ig sera. *Nature* **251**:63–64.

65. Feldmann M and Basten A. (1972). Cell interactions in the immune response *in vitro*. IV. Comparison of the effects of antigen-specific and allogeneic thymus-derived cell factors. *J Exp Med* **136**:722–736.

66. Feldmann M. (1974). T cell suppression *in vitro*. II. Nature of specific suppressive factor. *Eur J Immunol* **4**:667–674.

67. Takemori T and Tada T. (1975). Properties of antigen-specific suppressive T cell factor in the regulation of the antibody response of the mouse. I. *In vivo* activity and immunochemical characterizations. *J Exp Med* **142**:1241–1253.

68. Boyse E, Myazawa M, Aoki T and Old L. (1968). Ly-A and Ly-B: Two systems of lymphocyte isoantigens in the mouse. *Proc Roy Soc Ser B* **170**:175.

69. Boyse E, Itakura K, Stockert E, *et al.* (1971). Ly-C: A third locus specifying alloantigens expressed only on thymocytes and lymphocytes. *Transplantation* **11**:351.

70. Kisielow P, Hirst J, Shiku H, *et al.* (1975). Ly antigens as markers for functionally distinct subpopulations of thymus-derived lymphocytes of the mouse. *Nature* **253**:219–220.

71. Cohen L and Howe M. (1973). Synergism between subpopulations of thymus-derived cells mediating the proliferative and effector phases of the mixed lymphocyte reaction. *PNAS, USA* **70**:2707–2710.

72. Cantor H and Boyse E. (1975). Functional subclasses of T lymphocytes bearing different Ly antigens: I. The generation of functionally distinct T cell subclasses is a differentiative process independent of antigen. *J Exp Med* **141**:1376–1389.
73. Cantor H and Boyse E. (1975). Functional subclasses of T lymphocytes bearing different Ly antigens: II. Cooperation Between Subclasses of Ly+ Cells in the Generation of Killer Activity. *J Exp Med* **141**:1390–1399.
74. Cantor H, Shen F and Boyse E (1976). Separation of T helper cells from T suppressor cells expressing different Ly components. II. Activation by Antigen: after Immunization, Antigen-Specific Suppressor and Helper Activities are Mediated by Distinct T-Cell Subclasses. *J Exp Med* **143**:1391–1401.
75. Murphy D, Herzenberg L, Okumura K, *et al.* (1976). A new I subregion marked by a locus (Ia-4) controlling surface determinants on suppressor T lymphocytes. *J Exp Med* **144**:699–712.
76. Tada T, Taniguchi M and David C. (1976). Properties of the antigen-specific suppressive T cell factor in the regulation of antibody response of the mouse. *J Exp Med* **144**:713–725.
77. Benacerraf B. (1978). A hypothesis to relate the specificity of T-lymphocytes and the activity of I region-specific Ir genes in macrophages and B lymphocytes. *J Immunol* **120**:1809–1812.

2 From Activities to Molecules: The Interleukins

Lymphocyte-Conditioned Media (Ly-CM)

The only *in vitro* assays available to identify the molecules responsible for the various activities that had been found in leukocyte-conditioned media monitored one of three functions; proliferation, antibody formation and cell-mediated cytotoxicity. Thus, it is noteworthy that in 1976 Janet Plate described a T cell-derived soluble activity that could replace helper T cells in the generation of cytolytic T lymphocytes (CTL), a new function.[1] However, she could not differentiate the CTL helper activity from Blastogenic factor assayed by proliferation, or the TRFs assayed by the generation of AFCs as described by Schimpl and Wecker or Taussig and Monro. Thus, based upon the assays used, by 1976 there were descriptions of a myriad of soluble activities in lymphocyte-conditioned media.

At about the same time, several investigators used repetitive alloantigen stimulation to maintain antigen-reactive cells in culture for longer than just a few days. There were varied reports of success ranging from 3–4 weeks to several months. H. Robson McDonald, working with Jean Charles Cerottini and Theodore Brunner, first reported in 1974 that it was possible to maintain murine CTL in culture using weekly or bi-weekly repetitive alloantigen stimulation for periods as long as two months.[2] Erik Svedmyr reported similar findings using human MLCs in 1975.[3] He was successful in maintaining cells for as long as four months by re-stimulating them bi-weekly. Also in 1975, Zivi Ben-Sasson working with Ira Green showed that it was possible to use soluble protein antigen-pulsed adherent cell monolayers to repetitively stimulate guinea pig lymphocytes for

31

periods of 2–5 weeks.[4] Gunther Dennert used similar procedures and repetitive murine MLCs to continuously culture alloreactive cells for as long as nine months in 1976.[5] Accordingly, in a period of just a few years, investigators operating under the dogma that specific antigen activated the proliferation of T cells, found that T cells could be repetitively antigen-stimulated and cultured for prolonged periods. However, none of these investigators mentioned soluble mitogenic factors as responsible.

Against this background, a 1976 report by Doris Morgan and co-workers serendipitously found that conditioned media from PHA-stimulated human lymphocytes promoted the long-term culture of human bone marrow T cells for periods as long as 13 weeks.[6] These investigators had been searching for a growth factor that could facilitate the growth of human acute myeloid leukemia cells (AML), and had used PHA-stimulated lymphocyte-conditioned media (LyCM), because it had previously been reported to be a source for Granulocyte Colony Stimulating Activity (G-CSA).[7] Because they had used bone marrow as the cell source for their cultures, which was known to contain immature precursor T cells, it was not clear whether the cells grown were immature or mature T cells, in that they had not demonstrated any physiological mature T cell functions.[8]

Initially, it looked as though Morgan's cultured cells might be Epstein-Barr Virus (EBV)-transformed B cells. However, experiments using fresh rather than PHA-stimulated Ly-CM could not support long-term T cell growth, and further tests indicated that >95% of the cells formed Erythrocyte rosettes (E-rosettes) with SRBCs, which was the only marker known at the time for human T cells.[9] Moreover, tests for myeloid markers were negative. Because PHA was a known T cell mitogen, the most plausible hypothesis was that the PHA in the Ly-CM itself was responsible. However, the use of fresh media + PHA could not support long-term T cell growth either. Accordingly, the default hypothesis was that a soluble mitogenic factor or activity secreted into the Ly-CM by the PHA-stimulated cells might be responsible. In this regard, one is reminded of Peter Nowell's conjecture that perhaps PHA stimulation caused the cells to secrete a soluble factor that actually provided the growth signal for the cells,[10] as well as Blastogenic Factor.[11,12]

Additional experiments were performed using peripheral blood mononuclear cells (PBMCs) rather than bone marrow cells as a source of the long-term T cell cultures, thereby excluding the possibility that the cells selected for growth in the Ly-CM were exclusively immature T cell precursors. For these studies, we collaborated with Morgan's group,[9] and established that activation of the cultured T cells with T cell mitogens resulted in the production of IFN activity, an accepted functional characteristic of mature T cells as compared with immature T cells.[9] Even so, because the long-term T cell cultures were initiated and maintained using PHA-stimulated Ly-CM, the role played by the PHA vs. any putative growth factor was unclear. Also, because PHA was known to activate polyclonal T cell proliferation, it was impossible to probe for any antigen-specific functions of the cultured cells.

Cytolytic T Lymphocyte Lines (CTLL)

At the time, we had already established systems using murine splenocytes to generate CTL capable of lysing both allogeneic and syngeneic leukemia cells in 1977.[13] First, we found that if we performed repetitive mixed tumor lymphocyte cultures (MTLC), we could enhance the generation of CTL as much as 100-fold. Then, with secondary but not primary allogeneic MTLC, it was possible to generate short-term T cell growth and differentiation to CTL capable of lysing both allogeneic and syngeneic leukemia cells. To explain our results, we speculated that the strong stimulation afforded by the histocompatibility antigens may have produced an allogeneic effect factor (AEF), similar to that found to enhance T–B cell interaction in the generation of AFCs.[14] We also postulated that by using allogeneic leukemia cells as stimulators, we might generate several different clones of cells, some reactive with alloantigens and some reactive with syngeneic tumor-specific antigens. This interpretation was compatible with the findings of Zinkernagel and Doherty, in that presumably the tumor-specific antigen could be expressed either as a part of the self MHC encoded molecule, i.e. altered self, or it could be distinct from the self MHC, requiring two TCRs for recognition. However, the nature of the T cell antigen recognition structure(s) was still an enigma.

Given the findings of Morgan and co-workers, we speculated that it might be possible to create tumor antigen-specific long-term cytolytic T cell cultures using Ly-CM. Because Concanavalin-A (Con-A) was known to be a better mitogen for murine cells than PHA, we prepared Con-A T cell supernatants (which later was referred to by some as CATSUP), and seeded CTL derived from allogeneic repetitive MTLCs using Friend Leukemia Virus (FLV)-transformed leukemia cells, in the hope that functional CTL could be maintained with the Ly-CM. This was considered a long shot, because the immunological dogma indicated that only specific antigen would be able to promote T cell proliferation. However, the very first experiments worked beautifully, and the first antigen-specific, long-term Cytolytic T Lymphocyte Lines (CTLL) were reported in 1977.[15]

At the time of this report, the CTLL had been in continuous culture for 22 weeks, and their allogeneic as well as syngeneic tumor cell cytolytic activity had increased >10-fold. The cells required Ly-CM derived from Con-A-stimulated normal splenocytes, while fresh media + Con-A could not support long-term growth, thereby suggesting that the Ly-CM contained an obligatory growth factor. We speculated that one of the important issues that could now be approached was the molecular nature of the growth factor activity in the Ly-CM, using the long-term CTLL as target cells in a bioassay. In addition, we also speculated that these long-term CTLL might also be useful in adoptive therapy for leukemias, since they were cytolytic for virus non-virus producer leukemia cells, which were the most analogous to human leukemia cells.

The T Cell Growth Factor Bioassay

Prior to the development of the CTLL, in 1977 Torgny Fredrickson and I had developed and reported a microassay for quantifying erythropoietin (EPO), using mouse fetal liver cells (FLC) as the target cells, which are composed of a large proportion of EPO-responsive erythroid precursor cells.[16,17] This assay was based on the fact that erythroid precursor cells proliferate and differentiate into hemoglobin-producing cells under the influence of EPO. Thus, we found that EPO exerted a concentration-dependent increase in tritiated thymidine (^{3}H-TdR) and radiolabeled iron (^{59}Fe) incorporation into erythroid precursor cells with a peak reaction detectable after only 24 hours of culture in microwells. The principles of the assay were adapted from interferon bioassays, which routinely employed doubling dilution titrations, and comparison of the 50% Effective Concentrations (EC_{50}) using probability analysis (Probit Analysis).[18] The rapidity of this assay, requiring only an overnight culture, together with the capacity to readily quantify the EPO concentrations was novel at the time, and allowed us to perform adsorption experiments with FLCs, which suggested that EPO interacted with cells by means of cell surface receptors.

Accordingly, once we had developed CTLL, it was natural to adapt the EPO microassay for the quantification of the growth factor in Ly-CM that was critical for the continuous CTLL proliferation. The quantitative microassay that we developed and reported in 1978 was a first for lymphokines activities, in that previous bioassays had only scored the presence or absence of a particular activity.[19] We coined the term T Cell Growth Factor (TCGF) to designate that this activity was distinctive by its capacity to mediate the long-term growth of the CTLL. The ability to quantify the TCGF activity allowed us to perform experiments on the biological characteristics of this activity for the first time. For example, we found that TCGF activity could be quantitatively depleted from Ly-CM by both mitogen-stimulated lymphocytes and the CTLL, but not by fresh lymphocytes. Moreover, only T-cell mitogens such as PHA and Con-A or alloantigens could elicit TCGF activity, B-cell mitogens such as LPS being inactive in this regard. In addition, the removal of T cells from splenocyte or PBMC populations markedly reduced their capacity for production of TCGF activity. However, as we noted, this did not rule out the involvement of other cells, especially macrophages, in TCGF production. We noted that similar T-cell factors, such as those reported to enhance the generation of lymphoid blast cells, AFCs, or CTLs could very well be similar to or identical with TCGF, but there was no way to distinguish between these various activities. Thus, we closed our report with, "*It is our hope that the bioassay described in this report will be of use in future experimentation to approach the isolation, characterization, and purification of TCGF and similar factors*".[19]

The new quantitative TCGF microassay was helpful immediately in regard to whether the TCGF activity also had T-cell differentiative activity that facilitated the generation of CTL. In a series of experiments reported in 1978, we established unequivocally that *"TCGF amplifies the generation of cytotoxic T cells.... Depletion of TCGF from* (allogeneic) *MTLC depressed both the number and cytolytic activity of cells generated, whereas addition of TCGF to MTLC enhanced both of these parameters."*[20] Just like the EPO effect on FLCs, which leads to both the proliferation of erythroid precursors and their differentiation into RBCs monitored by the uptake of ^{59}Fe into hemoglobin molecules, TCGF promoted both the proliferation and differentiation of CTL progenitor T cells.

The TCGF bioassay also allowed us to test Ly-CM derived from various species. It was found that mouse CTLL cells could also be maintained in Ly-CM from rat and man, but human T cells could not respond to mouse or rat TCGF. Thus, we could use the mouse CTLL bioassay to quantify the TCGF activity in human Ly-CM, so that we could optimize human TCGF production. This led us immediately to the creation of the first long-term antigen-specific human CTLLs, which we reported in 1978.[21] These human CTLL were very similar, if not identical to the murine CTLL, so that these experiments confirmed our murine studies, and by extending the phenomenon to the human, they underscored the biological generality of the continuous culture of antigen-specific functional T cells. These data also prompted us to predict that *"Such cells will undoubtedly prove useful for studies on the mechanism of LMC, and for characterization of T-cell antigen receptors and* (other) *T-cell surface markers."* We also speculated that human tumor-specific CTLL might conceivably be used for adoptive immunotherapy for cancer. In addition, it seemed reasonable to assume that it should be possible to generate functional helper and putative suppressor T-cell lines, which *"may provide a new means for the study of both the mechanism and regulation of T-cell mediated immunity."*

Murine Monoclonal Cytolytic T Cells

To move beyond descriptive T cell biology, it was necessary to reduce the tremendous complexity and heterogeneity of T cell populations to the progeny of a single T cell, so that it would be possible to fulfill Burnet's prediction that, *"Only by the use of a pure clone technique of tissue culture, which allows mesenchymal cells to retain full functional activity, would we be likely to find an answer* (to the Clonal Selection Hypothesis)."[22] Thus, following the lead of those who had employed repetitive alloantigen stimulation to generate long-term cultures of T cells, in 1978 Garrison Fathman and Hans Hengartner attempted to use repetitive Mixed Leukocyte Cultures (MLC) to develop T cell clones.[23] Unfortunately, their cultured cells lost their antigen-specific cytolytic capacities so that they could not demonstrate clonality. Marcus Nabholz and co-workers also in 1978 tried to generate cytolytic clones of alloreactive cells using colony formation in soft agar.[24] However, they too could not demonstrate monoclonal cytolytic function, and both groups had no way to expand any cells that they had isolated beyond repetitive MLC.

Because our long-term Cytotoxic T Lymphocyte Lines (CTLL) had been generated against allogeneic leukemia cells, and had demonstrable alloantigen cytolytic specificity as well as syngeneic tumor-specific cytolytic specificity, in 1979 after 17 weeks of continuous culture in T Cell Growth Factor (TCGF; IL-2) we cloned the cells using TCGF in liquid suspension culture in microtiter plates.[25] We hypothesized that we should obtain some clones with only alloreactivity and others with tumor-specific reactivity. Cells were seeded by limiting dilution at 0.3–0.1 cells/well, so that by Poisson statistics the probability that wells would be seeded with more than one cell was <0.05. Remarkably, the calculated plating efficiency ranged from 67%–100%. Of 24 clones tested for cytolytic activity against allogeneic vs. syngeneic leukemia cells, 10 (42%) specifically only lysed the allogeneic targets, four clones (17%) lysed only the syngeneic targets, six clones (25%) lysed both allogeneic and syngeneic targets, and four (17%) were not cytolytic for either target. The cytolytic pattern of the clones remained constant over several weeks of culture, and to further prove clonality, one clone was selected and subcloned: all subclones demonstrated identical cytolytic activity. This was the first report that it was possible to derive true monoclonal cytolytic T cells. We concluded that, *"detailed studies of the phenotypic and functional characteristics of monospecific, homogeneous, cytolytic T lymphocytes will now be possible."*[25]

The methods detailed in this first paper regarding T cell cloning[25] were rapidly taken up and reproduced by everyone interested in generating their own antigen-specific T cell clones. Noteworthy among one of the first confirmatory reports using our methods to expand and grow large quantities of clonal progeny, was the creation of a clone cytolytic for a male-specific minor histocompatibility antigen (H-Y) by Harald von Boehmer and colleagues.[26] Von Boehmer's group immunized female mice with male H-Y+ splenocytes, then activated the female splenocytes by repetitive MLC *in vitro*, followed by growth in soft agar containing Con-A T cell supernatant (CATSUP) until microscopic colonies (20–30 cells) could be observed, picked and expanded in Lymphocyte Conditioned Medium (Ly-CM). Thus, the introduction of the growth-promoting properties of the Ly-CM were critical, in that they enabled the continuous propagation and expansion of the progeny so that the cells could be characterized and proved to be derived from a single cell. Also, when these investigators re-cloned the original cell line to prove clonality, they used our limiting dilution method rather than colony formation in soft agar. Limiting dilution cloning is much simpler and very efficient.

Monoclonal Antibodies and Human T Cell Surface Molecules (T3, T4, T8)

The other major advance that occurred during the 1970s was George Kohler's and Cesar Milstein's 1975 report of the development of methods to create somatic cell hybrids (hybridomas) using mouse plasmacytoma cells and B cells from splenocytes from mice immunized with SRBCs, thereby generating monoclonal antibodies with defined antigen specificity.[27] This advance was truly revolutionary, because for the first time hybridomas could be generated and expanded to produce unlimited quantities of individual antibodies that could be used for a myriad of research purposes. In particular, the hybridoma technology brought the study of human immune responses into the forefront, because it was simple to immunize mice with human cells and molecules to produce specific MoAbs, whereas obviously, mouse cells and molecules were not immunogenic for mice. Not until almost a decade later were

MoAbs raised against murine antigens, by immunizing either rats or hamsters to produce B cell fusion partners for murine plasmacytomas.

One of the first breakthroughs was from Ellis Reinherz and co-workers who reported in 1979 the separation of functional subsets of human T cells by a monoclonal antibody.[28] Using a MoAb designated OKT4 raised against human peripheral T cells,[29] Reinherz and coworkers found that the MoAb reacted with ~60% of peripheral human T cells, while it was unreactive with human B cells, null cells and macrophages. Separation of human peripheral T cells into OKT4+ and OKT4- subsets, followed by testing for proliferative responses to T cell mitogens and antigens, indicated that both subsets were responsive to T cell mitogens, but that most of the proliferative capacity of T cells resided in the OKT4+ population. Even more remarkable, after an MLC, most of the cytolytic activity was attributable to the OKT4- subset, while the OKT4+ subset appeared to provide helper activity for Cytolytic T Lymphocyte (CTL) generation, as we had shown for TCGF.[20] As noted by the authors, the OKT4 MoAb appeared to recognize the human T cell subset equivalent to that defined by murine Ly1 alloantisera reported by Kisielow[30] and independently by Cantor and Boyse.[31] Additional experiments by Reinherz and colleagues affirmed that the OKT4+ subset provided "help" for the generation of antibody forming cells (AFCs) from human B cells whereas the OKT4- subset did not.[32] However, the mechanism(s) whereby the helper T cells (Th) promoted both the generation of CTL and AFCs remained to be defined.

MoAbs that recognized the reciprocal, cytolytic/suppressor subset, OKT5/8 (subsequently renamed CD8)·were reported soon thereafter in 1980 by Reinherz and co-workers.[33] This MoAb was found to react with the human homologue of the murine determinant Ly2, recognized by the murine alloantisera. By using MoAbs, instead of alloantisera, and the new, very sensitive technique of flow cytometry,[34] in 1980 Leonard Herzenberg's group found the mouse Ly1 alloantigens are expressed on all T cells to varying amounts, so that a reciprocal marker for the mouse helper/inducer T cell subset, like human T4, was lacking. Actually, a MoAb that recognized the murine homologue of human T4 was only generated four years later in 1983 by Deno Dialynas working with Frank Fitch and his group.[35]

Human Monoclonal Cytolytic T Cells

In the interval, in 1982 Reinherz's group had already derived both T4⁺ and T5/8⁺ human alloreactive cytolytic T cell clones. By stimulating peripheral blood mononuclear cells (PBMCs) with an epstein-barr virus (EBV)-transformed B cell line in an MLC, T cell clones were obtained using both colony formation in soft agar and limiting dilution, followed by expansion in Ly-CM containing TCGF. They found that the T5/8⁺ clones were reactive against HLA-A and B antigens (MHC class I), while the T4⁺ clones were reactive against Immune-associated (Ia) antigens (MHC class II).[36] Thus, whatever the nature of the T Cell antigen Receptor (TCR), these cloned T cells specifically recognized either the serologically defined HLA-encoded molecules or I-region encoded molecules on the surface of alloantigen presenting cells, but not both. It is noteworthy that of fifteen T8⁺ clones tested, all exhibited a high level of cytotoxicity against the stimulating alloantigen, while only two of seven T4⁺ clones tested exhibited cytotoxicity. However, it is equally noteworthy that T4⁺ clones could become cytolytic, indicating that there was not a strict delineation between the functions of human T4⁺ vs. T8⁺ clones, such as helper vs. cytolytic that had been defined by studying T cell populations.

Of equal or even greater importance for understanding T cell antigen recognition was Reinherz's 1980 report that the OKT3 MoAb blocked antigen-induced T cell proliferation.[37] By comparison with the T cell subset MoAbs, this MoAb recognized all peripheral T cells as well as ~10% of thymocytes with high immunoreactivity by flow cytometry. In this regard, reminiscent of Peter Nowell's 1961 experiments showing that glucocorticoids suppressed phytohemagglutinin (PHA)-induced lymphocyte blastogenesis and mitosis only if added soon after PHA,[38] OKT3 was only maximally suppressive when added at the initiation of antigen stimulation. By comparison, several other MoAbs had no suppressive effects whatsoever, including OKT1, OKT4, OKT5/8, anti-Ia and anti-beta-2-microglobulin. Reinherz interpreted their findings as: *"Both the appearance of this antigen in intrathymic ontogeny and its critical role in T cell function suggests that the T3 molecule is related to an important antigen recognition receptor."*

In this regard, it is noteworthy that Reinherz's group had used the reciprocal anti-T4 and anti-T5/8 MoAbs, together with anti-T3 to show that the majority of human thymocytes were positive for both T4 and T5/8 (i.e. "double positive"), while <10% of thymocytes were T3+, and these cells were only positive for either T4 or T5/8 expression, but not both (i.e. "single positive").[39] It was not until five years later in 1985 that the first murine T3 molecule was identified,[40] so that Reinherz's findings were finally confirmed in the mouse. Of note, in 1984 the First International Cluster of Differentiation (CD) Workshop nomenclature committee was so compelled by the wealth of data on T3, T4 and T8 that these molecules were named CD3, CD4 and CD8 accordingly (http://www.uniprot.org/docs/cdlist).[41] These workshops were very important, because they allowed investigators to test their MoAbs to ascertain whether they were reactive with known CDs or whether new CDs should be designated. Today there are more than 350 designated CD markers, and the list is still growing (http://en.wikipedia.org/wiki/Cluster_of_differentiation).

The Interleukins

While these articles focused on human antigen-specific recognition by T cells, my team was focused on the antigen *nonspecific* nature of the activities of soluble factors involved in the antigen-specific adaptive T cell response. When we submitted our findings describing the TCGF bioassay,[19] one of the reviewers asked how we could discriminate TCGF from macrophage-derived Lymphocyte Activating Factor (LAF).[42] The LAF bioassay depended upon demonstrating enhanced proliferative activity of macrophage supernatants on murine thymocytes activated by PHA and cultured at high density (10^7 cells/mL) for several days.[43] Also, as already noted, it was well known that purified T cells were markedly less responsive to T cell mitogenic lectins than cell populations containing both lymphocytes and macrophages.[44] Accordingly, in 1980 we tested for Con-A-induced TCGF production by purified T cells compared with unpurified splenocytes, and found that TCGF production was reduced by ~85%, as determined by the TCGF quantitative assay.[45] Although adherent cells alone produced no detectable

TCGF activity, reconstitution of purified T cells with small numbers of adherent cells completely restored TCGF production.[46] By comparison, thymocytes did not produce detectable TCGF.

These findings indicated that adherent cells and mature T cells must somehow cooperate upon mitogenic lectin stimulation to produce TCGF. Furthermore, they suggested that perhaps the limiting factor in thymocyte TCGF production was a relative deficiency of adherent cells. However, as shown by Reinherz, only ~10% of thymocytes were mature, and in 1979 we reported that only the cortisol-resistant thymocytes, which comprised ~10% of thymocytes, were capable of producing TCGF.[47] Therefore, perhaps the majority of thymocytes, being immature simply could not produce TCGF. However, we still could not be sure which cell type actually produced TCGF, macrophage or mature T cell. Thus, in collaboration with Joost Oppenheim's group, we tested his purified preparation of human macrophage-derived LAF and his purified preparation of human lymphocyte-derived mitogenic activity, and found that the LAF had no activity in the TCGF assay, whereas the lymphocyte-derived activity was positive in both the LAF assay and the TCGF bioassay. Also, our TCGF preparation scored positively in both the thymocyte LAF assay and the CTLL TCGF assay. We presented our findings together at the Second International Lymphokine Workshop held in Ermatingen Switzerland, in May 1979, and for the first time it was appreciated by all investigators present that by using the TCGF bioassay it was possible to discriminate between monocyte/macrophage-derived LAF and lymphocyte-derived TCGF.[48] These findings electrified the conference and led to many late-night discussions as to how to interpret the fact that LAF and TCGF were separable, at least functionally.

Even so, it was still unclear as to how LAF could be mitogenic for thymocytes and purified T cells, but not mitogenic for CTLL. Therefore, in additional 1980 experiments, we showed that purified LAF preparations prepared from lipopolysaccharide (LPS)-induced human PBMCs prompted cloned murine lymphoma cells to produce TCGF in a LAF-concentration-dependent manner.[49] Thus, it appeared that LAF promoted TCGF production and that both LAF and TCGF comprised *"a bimodal amplification system for the T cell immune response."* Moreover, because LAF was routinely produced from macrophages via stimulation by LPS, a common immunological adjuvant, these data indicated that this could explain how adjuvants like LPS functioned to markedly amplify immune responses. In still other experiments in collaboration with Oppenheim and Lawrence Lachman, using their purified human and murine LAF preparations, respectively, we confirmed these findings and extended them by showing that glucocorticoids inhibited LAF production from macrophages, and consequently the LAF-induced proliferation of thymocytes, but did not suppress the TCGF-induced proliferation of thymocytes.[50] All of these data were included in a 1980 review that summarized our progress and proposed a new model for T cell activation that explained many of the experimental findings that had been enigmatic.[45]

Accordingly, because LAF and TCGF were clearly distinguishable functionally by the TCGF assay, and because LAF was mitogenic for thymocytes and purified T cells *because* it enhanced T cell TCGF production, these data provided the scientific rationale for the interleukin nomenclature. Thus, subsequent to the Ermatingen Workshop, a proposal was circulated and signed by most of those investigators working in the field of antigen-nonspecific T cell proliferation and helper factors. It was proposed that LAF be renamed interleukin-1 (IL-1) because it worked upstream, and TCGF be named Interleukin-2 receptor (IL-2), because it was downstream of LAF activity.[51] The term *interleukin* was coined to designate that messages were passed between *(inter)* leukocytes *(leukin)*. Like the complement field, we anticipated additional interleukins yet to be discovered. Now, in 2017 there are 39 interleukins, which constitutes the "modern" nomenclature for these newly discovered hormone-like molecules.

By comparison, identification of the molecule(s) responsible for antigen-specific helper and suppressor activities first described in Chapter 1 still had not progressed beyond their original descriptions, i.e. the removal of the activities by antigen-bound Sepharose and immunoaffitinity columns of Ia alloantisera. As chairman of the session on antigen-specific factors, Marc Feldmann summarized the lack of progress in defining the biochemical natures of the various antigen-specific helper and suppressor factors at the Second International Lymphokine Workshop in 1979: "*All we can say at this moment is that there is probably a family of helper and suppressor factors.*"[52]

The First Interleukin Molecule, IL-2

Although the new nomenclature in many ways simplified soluble antigen-nonspecific mitogenic factors by placing them into two categories, one macrophage-derived and the other lymphocyte-derived, the nomenclature was premature, because neither IL-1 nor IL-2 activities had been purified to homogeneity and ascribed to single, individual molecules. Thus, by 1980 it was clear to all in the field that the next step was purification.

Most investigators chose to attempt to identify and purify the molecules responsible for murine mitogenic activities.[53-57] An illustrative 1979 report by James Watson in collaboration with Lucien Aarden, Jennifer Shaw and Verner Paetkau focused on the purification of 200 mL of supernatant from 10 Balb/c spleens (~10^9 splenocytes) activated with Con-A for 18 hours in media supplemented with 1% Fetal Calf Serum (FCS).[58] After ammonium sulfate precipitation of the proteins, the sample was subjected to molecular gel filtration, ion exchange chromatography, and isoelectric focusing. After each step, fractions were monitored for activity in three distinct assays; (1) T cell replacing activity for splenocyte AFCs; (2) Con-A-induced thymocyte mitogenesis-the LAF assay; and (3) induction of thymocyte alloantigen-specific CTL. These investigators found that fractionation of the Ly-CM by these methods yielded results that indicated "*the molecules responsible for biological activity in each assay system show identical behavior upon gel filtration, ion-exchange chromatography, and isoelectric focusing.*"[58]

By gel filtration, the activities corresponded in size to molecules from 30–40 kDa, and when applied to an ion-exchange column eluted with a salt gradient from 0.05–0.5 M ammonium acetate (pH 7.6), with identical activities in both the thymocyte LAF and AFC assays. By comparison, when monitored by isoelectric focusing (IEF), there was considerable heterogeneity in pI in the broad range of pH 4–5. As already mentioned, both macrophage-derived mitogenic factors (i.e. LAF) and putative T cell-derived mitogenic factors (i.e. TCGF, Thymocyte Stimulating Factor, TSF, T cell Replacing Factor, TRF) could not be discriminated by these bioassays. Because the target cells used, i.e. thymocytes and splenocytes, were heterogeneous, when fractions of Ly-CM derived from heterogeneous producer cells containing both macrophages and lymphocytes (and both B cells and T cells), it was impossible to dissect the contributions of one cell and molecule vs. another, and whether the target cells of a given activity in turn released an additional activity that was detected by the assay. Thus, it was truly GIGO (Garbage-In-Garbage-Out).

Also, the Ly-CM was produced in media containing 1% Fetal Calf Sera (FCS). Accordingly, it is important to calculate that 1% = 1 gm protein/dL = 10 mg/mL of FCS proteins in the Ly-CM. These investigators estimated that their cytokine activities were present in the Ly-CM at concentrations $\sim 10^{-9}$ M, which at molecular sizes of ~ 35 kDa = 35 ng/mL. Therefore, the cytokine activities were produced in media with a million-fold excess of FCS proteins vs. cytokine proteins. In fact, as we were to learn subsequently, TCGF is active at concentrations in the pg/mL range, so that by using 1% FCS to make the Ly-CM, the FCS proteins were a billion-fold in excess of the cytokine proteins. This made the purification of the FCS proteins away from the cytokine proteins essentially impossible. Also, because the cytokine protein(s) were present in infinitesimal amounts, it meant that to be successful, one needed to begin with very large quantities of Ly-CM. If the cytokine was present at 150 pg/mL = 10 pM, then 200 mL of Ly-CM contained only 30 ng of cytokine protein. This was definitely not enough to quantify using any of the available protein assays, such as the colorimetric Bradford assay, which requires > 1 µg protein.[59] Accordingly, even given 100% recovery of starting material, one would need to start with at least 7 L of Ly-CM, which would equate to 350 mouse spleens, not just 10.

By comparison with these efforts, we elected to focus on the purification and characterization of molecules with human TCGF activity. Having solved the problem of target cell heterogeneity by using murine CTLL clones, we could be confident that any effects observed were mediated by direct interaction of the lymphokine with the target T cells themselves. We decided to focus on human TCGF because ultimately, we hoped to raise a murine MoAb reactive to the molecule(s), and because eventually we hoped to be able to use TCGF in the clinic. Others at the time favored the notion that a family of molecules would prove to have TCGF activity, based on the broad elution profiles from the molecular sieve and ion exchange columns, and from the multiple peaks observed after IEF. If true, when the molecules were separated, the activity discernable in the bioassay would be lost.

To approach the problem of serum proteins contaminating TCGF, we developed a system to produce TCGF in serum-free media from human PBMCs. To increase the amounts of starting material, we switched to human tonsil lymphocytes, because we could obtain $\sim 10^9$ cells from each tonsil, which was equal to the number of lymphocytes in a liter of blood. Thus, it was possible to generate 1 L of PHA-induced Ly-CM from each tonsil, culturing the cells at 1 × 10^6 cells/mL. Several liters of Ly-CM were pooled and concentrated >1,000-fold by filtration, then purified successively by gel filtration, isoelectric focusing and polyacrylamide gel electrophoresis (PAGE). We could show that the heterogeneity of charge that others had found examining murine Ly-CM could be eliminated by removal of sialic acid and by the inhibition of glycosylation. Thus, we could show that TCGF activity could be ascribed to a molecule with a single charge (pI = 8.2) and size (14–16,000 Mr), and that all of the apparent molecular heterogeneity was attributable to variable glycosylation and not due to multiple protein molecules with TCGF activity.[60] Thus, as reported for the first time in 1981, the TCGF biological activity could be ascribed to a single variably glycosylated protein.

The TCGF (IL-2) Receptor

Having thus reduced the apparent molecular heterogeneity of TCGF activity to a single molecule, and knowing the biochemical characteristics of TCGF, i.e. its size and pI, we produced biosynthetically radiolabeled TCGF by culturing cells with amino acids tagged with radioisotopes, and then purified the radiolabeled TCGF using gel filtration and isoelectric focusing, until we had a single radiolabeled band on SDS-PAGE detectable by fluorography.[61] By monitoring the TCGF activity using the bioassay, and by measuring the protein concentration of unlabeled purified TCGF by amino acid analysis and dye binding, we could assign our preparations a Specific Activity, i.e. U/μg protein, and knowing the molecular size (15.5 kDa) we could calculate the molar concentration of both labeled and unlabeled TCGF (i.e. CPM/pmole). Thus, for the first time, we could determine that TCGF was active in the pM range. Ultimately, repeated determinations yielded a dose-response in the range of 1–100 pM with an EC_{50} = 5–10 pM.

Because our radiolabeled TCGF preparations were homogeneous and contained no other radiolabeled molecules, in 1981 we reported classical radiolabeled ligand-binding assays.[61] Kinetic and equilibrium binding experiments revealed that unstimulated human PBMCs had detectable binding sites, on the order of ~200 sites/cell (lower limit of detection = 60 sites/cell), but that upon activation, either with mitogenic lectins or alloantigens, the number of detectable binding sites increased remarkably, ~50-fold, to ~10,000 sites/cell. Upon plotting the equilibrium binding data of human radiolabeled TCGF to human cells by the method of Scatchard,[62] we found a single class of high affinity binding sites, with an equilibrium dissociation constant (K_d) ~5–10 pM, whereas in murine activated T cells and CTLL, the K_d was ~20 pM. Of utmost importance, the concentrations of radiolabeled TCGF that bound to cells, and the concentrations of unlabeled TCGF that promoted T cell proliferation (EC_{50} = 1 U/mL = 5 pM) were essentially identical. Moreover, when several other growth factors and lymphokines were tested, only TCGF successfully competed for radiolabeled TCGF binding.

Soon after the publication of these data, I was contacted by Thomas Waldmann. Takashi Uchiyama from his group had raised a MoAb that only reacted with a human leukemia cell line that had been used for immunization of mice to produce hybridomas.[63,64] They speculated that their MoAb might recognize the TCGF receptor, since it did not react with normal resting T cells, but did react after the T cells were activated via mitogenic lectins or alloanigens. The very first experiments were definitive, in that the MoAb, subsequently called anti-Tac (for activated T cell), competed for radiolabeled TCGF binding in a concentration-dependent manner.[65] Also, anti-Tac precipitated a single glycoprotein of ~55 kDa from radiolabeled cell surface molecules. Accordingly, these 1982 experiments described the first MoAb reactive with an interleukin receptor.

These findings were very significant, because for the first time they indicated that the immune system, like all other systems in the body, is under endogenous control via hormone-like molecules. Hormones and receptors had already been classically defined by physiologists in the late 19th century[66] and early 20th century,[67] as substances secreted by cells that act to elicit a characteristic physiological response at very low concentrations, via interaction with high affinity with a cellular receptor. Thus, TCGF had these characteristics of a bonafide hormone, including stereospecificity, high affinity, and a finite number of binding sites that are consequently saturable.

Prior to these findings, the immune system was viewed as regulated entirely from without via environmental molecules (antigens), that when introduced were recognized by specific antigen receptors, which led to the proliferation and differentiation of the cells that then cleared the antigens. Thus, it was *taught* that the immune system was distinct and special, set apart from every other organ system, and was only aroused and regulated from a quiescent state by external forces, much like the nervous system senses changes in the environment, e.g. temperature, light, sound etc. Therefore, it was thought that once the system cleared the offending antigen, if there was no longer a driving external force, it returned to quiescence. Consequently, this dogma was overturned by the finding that antigen-specific T cell clonal expansion is regulated by an endogenous hormone-receptor system like other organ systems. It remained true that the introduction of antigen activates the immune system, but after antigen recognition there is an endogenous, endocrine-like molecular mechanism that drives the proliferation and differentiation of the cells that mediate the antigen clearance.

The concept that an endocrine mechanism is responsible for immunoregulation, instead of solely being antigen-regulated, necessarily invoked a way to turn off the IL-2/IL-2R interaction. Of course, logic dictated that clearance of the antigen should result in the removal of the TCR-directed signals that control the expression of IL-2 and its receptors. However, to be termed a true hormonal system, endocrinologists required evidence for a hormone-induced negative feedback regulation of either hormone production or receptor expression, or both. Accordingly, these questions would require additional time and experimental approaches.

The IL-2 cDNA, IL-2 Gene, IL-2 MoAbs, and Pure Homogeneous IL-2

The following year, 1983, was an important year for interleukins, especially IL-2. Tadatsugu Taniguchi's group took advantage of the rapid, specific and quantitative IL-2 bioassay to identify a cDNA encoding human IL-2 activity.[68] mRNA was isolated from the JURKAT human T leukemia cell line that had been found to produce IL-2 upon mitogenic lectin stimulation.[69,70] Using methods of hybrid selection of mRNA and translation in Xenopus laevis oocytes, followed by assay for TCGF activity using the CTLL-2 cells, a cDNA was identified that possessed TCGF activity. The cDNA specified 153 amino acids and a 20-amino acid hydrophobic leader signal sequence so that the mature secreted protein contained 133 residues, yielding a calculated molecular size of 15,420.5 Da, almost identical to the molecular size we estimated previously by SDS-PAGE of both native and radiolabeled TCGF (IL-2).[60,61] Once the cDNA encoding IL-2 had been identified, both Taniguchi, and ourselves, isolated genomic clones encoding the entire IL-2 gene.[71,72] The IL-2 gene spans 8 kb and is organized into 4 exons.

Although these genetic studies were informative as to the primary structure of the IL-2 molecule, and would eventually permit studies on the TCR complex regulation of IL-2 gene expression, they did not immediately lead to the availability of large amounts of pure IL-2 for additional biochemical, biological and immunological studies.

However, we had developed several MoAbs reactive with IL-2, which we used as immunoadsorbants to purify milligram quantities of homogeneous IL-2 protein.[73] Analysis of immunoaffinity purified IL-2 indicated that it eluted as a single peak from a reverse-phase high pressure liquid chromatography (HPLC), and migrated as a single size (15.5 kDa) on silver stained SDS-PAGE. Proof that there were no other contaminating proteins in the immunoaffinity purified preparations was obtained by amino terminal amino acid sequence analysis, which identified a single amino terminus, and the first 15 residues. Because this amino acid sequence was identical to that predicted from the IL-2 cDNA nucleotide base sequence, the data indicated agreement between the predicted cDNA and actual amino acid sequence analysis, and thus proving that a single molecule mediated IL-2 biological activity.

In addition to proving useful for the immunoaffinity purification of IL-2, the IL-2 MoAbs effectively neutralized both human and murine IL-2 activity, but were nonreactive with rat-derived IL-2. In addition, the neutralization of IL-2 could be competitively antagonized by an excess of IL-2. Moreover, the concentrations of IL-2 MoAbs that neutralized IL-2 in a 24-hour bioassay were identical to the MoAb concentrations that block radiolabeled IL-2 equilibrium binding, which came to a steady state within 15 minutes. These experimental results essentially proved that the MoAb neutralizing capacity depended upon IL-2 binding by the MoAbs, and not due to nonspecific interference with cellular metabolism in the bioassay, a problem that had misled other investigators attempting to generate IL-2-specific MoAbs.[74,75]

Additional experiments exploring the immunoaffinity adsorption characteristics of four distinct IL-2 MoAbs indicated that the single most important parameter is the association rate, and the temperature-dependence of both the association and dissociation rates.[76] Thus, as the association rate increases directly with temperature, we found that the most efficient immunoaffinity adsorption occurred at 37°C, while the washing and elution steps were best performed at 4°C. Moreover, the efficiency of immunoaffinity adsorption of separate MoAbs varied according to their association rates. We also used the

IL-2 MoAbs in 1986 to create the first immunoassay (ELISA) for an interleukin.[77] For these experiments radiolabeled IL-2 and radiolabeled IL-2 MoAbs were used to determine the reaction kinetics at each stage of the immunoassay. Noteworthy was the finding that reaction rates are retarded remarkably when performed in the solid-phase vs. solution, and are more rapid at 37°C than either 20°C or 4°C. These advances were paradigmatic for the uses of MoAbs raised against all the interleukins that followed.

References

1. Plate J. (1976). Soluble factors substitute for T-T-cell collaboration in the generation of T-killer lymphocytes. *Nature* **260**:329–331.
2. McDonald H, Engers H, Cerottini J and KT B. (1974). Generation of cytotoxic T lymphocytes *in vitro*. II. The effect of repeated exposure to alloantigens on the cytotoxic activity of long-term mixed leukocyte cultures. *J Exp Med* **140**:718–730.
3. Svedmyr E. (1975). Long-term maintenance *in vitro* of human T cells by repeated exposure to the same stimulator cells. *Scand. J Immunol* **4**:421–427.
4. Ben-Sasson S, Paul W, Shevach E and Green I. (1975). *In vitro* selection and extended culture of antigen-specific T lymphocytes. I. Description of selection procedure and initial characterization of selected cells. *J Exp Med* **142**:90–105.
5. Dennert G and De Rose M. (1976). Continuously proliferating T killer cells specific for H-2b targets: selection and characterization. *J Immunol* **116**:p1601–1606.
6. Morgan DA, Ruscetti FW and Gallo R. (1976). Selective *in vitro* growth of T lymphocytes from normal human bone marrows. *Science* **193**: 1007–1008.
7. Cline M and Golde D. (1974). Production of colony-stimulating activity by human lymphocytes. *Nature* **248**:703–704.
8. Morgan D. (1988). Forward. In *Interleukin 2*. K. Smith, editor. San Diego, CA: Academic Press, Inc. xvii–xi.
9. Ruscetti FW, Morgan DA and Gallo RC. (1977). Functional and morphologic characterization of human T cells continuously grown *in vitro*. *J Immunol* **119**:131–138.

10. Nowell PC. (1960). Phytohemagglutinin: An initiator of mitosis in cultures of normal human leukocytes. *Cancer Research* **20**:462–468.

11. Kasakura S and Lowenstein L. (1965). A factor stimulating DNA synthesis derived from the medium of leukocyte cultures. *Nature* **208**:794–795.

12. Gordon J and MacLean LD. (1965). A lymphocyte-stimulating factor produced *in vitro*. *Nature* **208**:795–796.

13. Gillis S and Smith K. (1977). *In vitro* generation of tumor-specific cytotoxic lymphocytes. Secondary allogeneic mixed tumor lymphocyte culture of normal murine spleen cells. *J Exp Med* **146**:468–482.

14. Amerding D and Katz D. (1974). Activation of T and B lymphocytes *in vitro*: II. Biological and biochemical properties of an allogeneic effect factor (AEF) active in triggering specific B lymphocytes. *J Exp Med* **140**:19–37.

15. Gillis S and Smith KA. (1977). Long term culture of tumour-specific cytotoxic T cells. *Nature* **268**:154–156.

16. Fredrickson TN, Smith KA, Cornell CJ, Jasmin C and McIntyre OR. (1977). The interaction of erythropoietin with fetal liver cells I. Measurement of proliferation by tritiated thymidine incorporation. *Exp Hematol* **5**:254–265.

17. Smith K, Fredrickson T, Mobraaten L and DeMaeyer E. (1977). The interaction of erythropoietin with fetal liver cells. II. Inhibition of the erythropoietin effect by interferon. *Exp Hemat* **5**:333–340.

18. Jordan G. (1972). Basis for the probit analysis of an interferon plaque reduction assay. *J Gen Virol* **14**:49–61.

19. Gillis S, Ferm MM, Ou W and Smith KA. (1978). T cell growth factor: parameters of production and a quantitative microassay for activity. *J Immunol* **120**:2027–2032.

20. Baker PE, Gillis S, Ferm MM and Smith KA. (1978). The effect of T cell growth factor on the generation of cytolytic T cells. *J Immunol* **121**:2168–2173.

21. Gillis S, Baker PE, Ruscetti FW and Smith KA. (1978). Long-term culture of human antigen-specific cytotoxic T cell lines. *J Exp Med* **148**:1093–1098.

22. Burnet FM. (1959). *The Clonal Selection Theory of Acquired Immunity*. Cambridge: Cambridge University Press.

23. Fathman C and Hengartner H. (1978). Clones of allreactive T cells. *Nature* 272.

24. Nabholz M, Engers H, Collavo D and North M editors. (1978). *Cloned T Cell Lines with Specific Cytolytic Activity*. New York: Springer-Verlag. 176 pp.

25. Baker PE, Gillis S and Smith KA. (1979). Monoclonal cytolytic T-cell lines. *J Exp Med* **149**:273–278.

26. von Boehmer H, Hengartner H, Nabholz M, Lernhradt W, Schreier M and Hass W. (1979). Fine specificity of a continuously growing killer cell clone specific for H-Y antigen. *Eur J Immunol* **9**:592–597.

27. Kohler G and Milstein C. (1975). Continuous culture of fused cells secreting antibody of predefined specificity. *Nature* **256**:495–499.

28. Reinherz EL, Kung PC, Goldstein G and Schlossman SF. (1979). Separation of functional subsets of human T cells by a monoclonal antibody. *Proc Natl Acad Sci USA* **76**:4061–4065.

29. Kung P, Goldstein G, Reinherz E and Schlossman S. (1979). Monoclonal antibodies defining distinctive human T cell surface antigens. *Science* **206**:347–349.

30. Kisielow P, Hirst J, Shiku H, Beverley P, Hoffman M, Boyse E and Oettgen H. (1975). Ly antigens as markers for functionally distinct subpopulations of thymus-derived lymphocytes of the mouse. *Nature* **253**:219–220.

31. Cantor H and Boyse E. (1975). Functional subclasses of T lymphocytes bearing different Ly antigens: I. The generation of functionally distinct T cell subclasses is a differentiative process independent of antigen. *J Exp Med* **141**:1376–1389.

32. Reinherz E, Kung P, Goldstein G and Schlossman S. (1979). Further characterization of the human inducer T cell subset defined by monoclonal antibody. *J Immunol* **123**:2894–2896.

33. Reinherz E, Kung P, Goldstein G and Schlossman S. (1980). A monoclonal antibody reactive with the human cytotoxic/suppressor T cell subset previously defined by a heteroantiserum termed TH2. *J Immunol* **124**:1301–1307.

34. Ledbetter J, Rouse R, Micklem H and Herzenberg L. (1980). T cell subsets defined by expression of Lyt1,2,3 and Thy1 antigens. Two parameter immunofluorescence and cytotoxicity analysis with monclonal antibodies modifies current views. *J Exp Med* **152**:280.

35. Dialynas D, Quan Z, Wall K, Pierres A, Quintans J, Loken M, Pierres M and Fitch F. (1983). Characterization of the murine T cell surface molecule, designated L3T4, identified by monoclonal antibody GK1.5: similarity to the human leu-3/T4 molecule. *J Immunol* **131**:2445–2451.

36. Meuer S, Schlossman S and Reinherz E. (1982). Clonal analysis of human cytolytic T lymphocytes: T4+ and T8+ effector T cells recognize products of different major histocompatibility regions. *Proc Natl Acad Sci USA* **79**:4395–4399.

37. Reinherz EL, Hussey RE and Schlossman SF. (1980). A monoclonal anti-body blocking human T cell function. *Eur J Immunol* **10**:758–762.

38. Nowell PC. (1961). Inhibition of human leukocyte mitosis by predni-solone *in vitro. Cancer Res* **21**:1518–1523.

39. Reinherz E, Kung P, Goldstein G, Levey R and Schlossman S. (1980). Discrete stages of intrathymic differentiation: analysis of normal thymo-cytes and leukemic lymphoblasts of T cell lineage. *Proc Natl Acad Sci USA* **77**:1588–1592.

40. van den Elsen P, Shepley B, Cho M and Terhorst C. (1985). Isolation and characterization of a cDNA clone encoding the murine homologue of the human 20K T3/T-cell receptor protein. *Nature* **314**:542–544.

41. Bernard A and Boumsell L. (1984). The clusters of differentiation (CD) defined by the First International Workshop on Human Leucocyte Differentiation Antigens. *Human Immunol* **11**:1–10.

42. Gery I and Waksman BH. (1972). Potentiation of the T-lymphocyte response to mitogens: The cellular source of potentiating mediators. *J Exp Med* **136**:143–155.

43. Gery I, Gershon RK and Waksman B. (1972). Potentiation of the T-lymphocyte response to mitogens I. The responding cell. *J Exp Med* **136**:128–142.

44. Oppenheim J, Leventhal B and Hersh E. (1968). The transformation of column-purified lymphocytes with nonspecific and specific antigenic stimuli. *J Immunol* **101**:262–270.

45. Smith KA. (1980). T-cell growth factor. *Immunol Rev* **51**:337–357.

46. Smith K, Baker P, Gillis S and Ruscetti F. (1980). Functional and molecu-lar characterization of T cell Growth Factor. *Mol Immunol* **17**:579–589.

47. Smith K, Gillis S and Baker P. (1979). The role of soluble factors in the regulation of T cell immune reactivity. In *The Molecular Basis of Immune Cell Function*. J. Kaplan, editor. Amsterdam, NL: Elsevier/North Holland Biomedical Press. 223–237.

48. Oppenheim J, Nortoff H, Greenhill A, Mathieson B, Smith K and Gillis S. (1980). Properties of human monocyte derived lymphocyte activating factor (LAF) and lymphocyte derived mitogenic factor (LMF). In *Biochemical Characterization of Lymphokines: Proceedings of the Second International Lymphokine Workshop*. A. de Weck, F. Kristensen, and M. Landy, editors. New York: Academic Press, Inc. 399–404.

49. Smith K, Gilbride K and Favata M. (1980). Lymphocyte activating factor promotes T cell growth factor production by cloned murine lymphoma cells. *Nature* **287**:853–855.

50. Smith KA, Lachman LB, Oppenheim JJ and Favata MF. (1980). The functional relationship of the interleukins. *J Exp Med* **151**:1551–1556.
51. Letter. (1979). Revised nomenclature for antigen-nonspecific T cell proliferation and helper factors. *J Immunol* **123**:2928–2929.
52. Feldmann M. (1980). Biochemical Characterization of Lymphokines. In *Second International Lymphokine Workshop*, A. De Weck, F. Kristensen, and M. Landy, editors. Ermatingen, Switzerland: Academic Press, p. 585.
53. Di Sabato G, Chen D and Erickson J. (1975). Production by murine spleen cells of an activity stimulating the PHA-responsiveness of thymus lymphocytes. *Cell Immunol* **17**:495–504.
54. Watson J. (1973). The role of humoral factors inthe initiation of *in vitro* primary immune responses. III. Characterization of factors that replace thymus-derived cells. *J Immunol* **111**:1301.
55. Farrar J, Simon P, Koopman W and Fuller-Bonar. (1978). Biochemical relationship of thymocyte mitogenic factor and factors enhancing humoral and cell-mediated immune responses. *J Immunol* **121**:1353.
56. Shaw J, Monticone V, Mills G and Paetkau V. (1978). Effects of costimulator on immune responses *in vitro*. *J Immunol* **120**:1974.
57. Shaw J, Monticone V and Paetkau V. (1978). Partial purification and molecular characterization of a lymphokine (costimulator) required for the mitogenic response of mouse thymocytes *in vitro*. *J Immunol* **120**:1967.
58. Watson J, Aarden L, Shaw J and Paetkau V. (1979). Molecular and quantitative analysis of helper T cell replacing factors on the induction of antigen-sensitive B and T lymphocytes. *J Immunol* **122**:1633–1638.
59. Bradford M. (1976). A rapid and sensitive method for the quantification of microgram quantities of protein utilizing the principle of protein-dye binding. *Anal Biochem* **72**:248.
60. Robb RJ and Smith KA. (1981). Heterogeneity of human T-cell growth factor(s) due to variable glycosylation. *Mol Immunol* **18**:1087–1094.
61. Robb RJ, Munck A and Smith KA. (1981). T cell growth factor receptors: Quantitation, specificity, and biological relevance. *J Exp Med* **154**:1455–1474.
62. Scatchard G. (1949). The attractions of proteins for small molecules and ions. *Ann NY Acad Sci* **51**:660–673.
63. Uchiyama T, Broder S and Waldmann TA. (1981). A monoclonal antibody (anti-Tac) reactive with activated and functionally mature human T cells. I. Production of anti-Tac monoclonal antibody and distribution of Tac (+) cells. *J Immunol* **126**:1393–1397.

64. Uchiyama T, Nelson DL, Fleisher TA and Waldmann TA. (1981). A monoclonal antibody (anti-Tac) reactive with activated and functionally mature human T cells. II. Expression of Tac antigen on activated cytotoxic killer T cells, suppressor cells, and on one of two types of helper T cells. *J Immunol* **126**:1398–1403.

65. Leonard WJ, Depper JM, Uchiyama T, Smith KA, Waldmann TA and Greene WC. (1982). A monoclonal antibody that appears to recognize the receptor for human T-cell growth factor; partial characterization of the receptor. *Nature* **300**:267–269.

66. Langley J. (1878). On the physiology of the salivary secretion. *J Physiol (Lond)* **1**:339–369.

67. Langley J. (1905). On the reaction of cells and nerve endings to certain poisons, chiefly as regards the reaction of striated muscle to nicotine and to curari. *J Physiol (Lond)* **33**:374–413.

68. Taniguchi T, Matsui H, Fujita T, Takaoka C, Kashima N, Yoshimoto R and Hamuro J. (1983). Structure and expression of a cloned cDNA for human interleukin-2. *Nature* **302**:305–310.

69. Gillis S and Watson J. (1980). Biochemical and biological characterization of lymphocyte regulatory molecules. *J Exp Med* **152**:1709–1719.

70. Kaplan J, Tilton J and Peterson WJ. (1975). Identification of T cell lymphoma tumor antigens on human T cell lines. *Am J Hematol* **1**: 219–227.

71. Fugita T, Takaoka C, Matsui H and Taniguchi T. (1983). Structure of the human interleukin-2 gene. *Proc Natl Acad Sci USA* **80**:7437–7441.

72. Holbrook NJ, Smith KA, Fornace AJ, Jr., Comeau CM, Wiskocil RL and Crabtree GR. (1984). T-cell growth factor: complete nucleotide sequence and organization of the gene in normal and malignant cells. *Proc Natl Acad Sci USA* **81**:1634–1638.

73. Smith KA, Favata MF and Oroszlan S. (1983). Production and characterization of monoclonal antibodies to human interleukin 2: strategy and tactics. *J Immunol* **131**:1808–1815.

74. Gillis S and Henney C. (1981). The biochemical and biological characterization of lymphocyte regulatory molecules. VI. Generation of a B cell hybridoma whose antibody product inhibits IL-2 activity. *J Immunol* **126**:1978–1983.

75. Stadler B, Berenstein E, Siraganian R and Oppenheim J. (1982). Monoclonal antibody against human interleukin-2 (IL-2). I. Purification of IL-2 for the production of monoclonal antibodies. *J Immunol* **128**:1620–1628.

76. Budd R and Smith KA. (1986). Interleukin 2 monoclonal antibody affinity adsorption: the critical role of binding kinetics for optimal immunoadsorption. *J Immunol Meth* **95**:237–248.
77. Budd R and Smith KA. (1986). Interleukin 2 immunoassay using monoclonal antibodies. *Biotechnology* **4**:983–986.

3 The Beginnings of Molecular Immunology

The T Cell Antigen Receptor (TCR) Complex Proteins

Having developed and propagated IL-2-dependent human T4$^+$ and T8$^+$ cytolytic T cell clones, Ellis Reinherz's group was in a unique position to identify the molecules responsible for T cell antigen recognition. Thus, in a seminal report, Reinherz and his group cracked the enigma of the molecular nature of the antigen recognition components of the TCR, and revealed the entire TCR complex for the first time in 1983.[1] Operating under Burnet's Clonal Selection Theory of Immunity, which led to their hypothesis that *"there must exist discriminative surface recognition structures that are unique to individual antigen-responsive T cell clones,"* Reinherz's group used one of their human T8$^+$ cytolytic T cell clones to immunize mice to produce murine hybridomas, and developed a screening strategy to select for clone-specific (clonotypic) MoAbs.

It was first important to determine whether the surface structures that the clone-specific MoAbs identified were involved in antigen recognition. Two such MoAbs were found to block both the specific cytotoxic function and antigen-induced proliferation of the immunizing T8$^+$ T cell clone. Also noteworthy, these MoAbs enhanced the proliferation of the T cell clone in response to IL-2. Moreover, the surface molecules defined by the MoAbs were linked to the T3 structure, but in contrast to T3 (Mr ~20 kDa), they precipitated two associated glycoproteins of apparent molecular weights of 49 and 43 kDa. Reinherz and his group interpreted their results in an understated, more British, than American fashion: *"It is likely that the*

59

clonotypic MoAbs define variable regions of the human T cell antigen receptor (on the T cell clone) *because they recognize clonotypic structures and inhibit antigen-specific function."*

Subsequently, to determine whether analogous receptor molecules could be found on other T cell clones of differing antigen specificity, MoAbs were generated against a T4⁺ cytolytic T cell clone.[2] Three MoAbs from ~600 hybridomas were selected, cloned and recloned by limiting dilution. Analysis of the molecular nature of the T4⁺ clone surface molecules recognized by all three antibodies yielded a 90 kDa molecule under non-reducing conditions, and two distinct bands, a ~51 kDa α-chain and 43 kDa β-chain under reducing conditions, thus very similar to the chains observed on the T8⁺ T cell clone. Also similar to the effects of the T8⁺ clone-specific MoAbs, the T4⁺ cytolytic clone-reactive MoAbs blocked alloantigen-specific cytolysis, as well as proliferation, and enhanced IL-2 induced proliferation. These findings supported the conclusions; *"that the basic subunit composition of the antigen receptors on cells derived from both the T4⁺ and T8⁺ human T cell subpopulations is similar. In contrast, recognition of class II or class I alloantigens by these subsets may be determined by the associative recognition structures T4 or T8, which are independent of Ti/T3."* Also, *"the wide distribution of the 20/25 kDa T3 glycoprotein and the ability of anti-T3 antibodies to inhibit antigen specific function of all clones suggest that T3 is a constant portion of the antigen receptor complex."*

Consistent with this view, the Reinherz group also derived a series of T4⁺ clones reactive with specific protein antigens, Ragweed Antigen E (RWAGE), and Tetanus Toxoid (TT).[3] Incubation of these clones with specific antigen together with autologous APCs and B cells resulted in the production of IgG. These T cell clones demonstrated a clear restriction for autologous class II MHC molecules. Immunization with one of the RAGWE-specific clones yielded one clonotypic MoAb from ~500 hybridomas. Biochemical analysis of immunoprecipitates showed a similar 90 kDa protein under nonreducing conditions and 52 kDa and 41 kDa under reducing conditions, along with the associated T3 20/25 kDa molecules.

Accordingly, for the first time Reinherz revealed for everyone the complete TCR complex utilized by both T cell subsets to recognize and react with antigen. Also, using both flow cytometry and radiolabeled quantitative clone-specific MoAb binding analysis, they found that both the clonotypic (Ti) and T3 structures to be expressed at a similar level on the cell surface, ~30–40,000 molecules/cell, whereas the density of T4 and T8 expressed by the clones was ~120,000–175,000 binding sites/cell, a 3-6–fold excess.[2] Other experiments showed that resting, freshly isolated T cells had equivalent densities of all three TCR complex structures, so that antigen or IL-2 activation was speculated to induce the enhanced levels of the accessory molecules T4 and T8.

Because T3 and clone-specific (Ti) structures appeared to be associated as they were expressed in equivalent densities and were co-modulated by their respective MoAbs, additional studies were performed to further explore this apparent non-covalent interaction. Having multiple T cell clones available, cell surface radiolabeled molecules could be immunoprecipitated with anti-T3 and analyzed by SDS-PAGE under reducing conditions.[4] In addition to T3 molecules of 20 and 25 kDa, two larger bands of ~49 and 43 kDa were observed from all clones tested. Also, two-dimensional SDS-PAGE analysis of the molecules precipitated with anti-T3 revealed two identical molecules with distinct pIs from the 25 kDa molecules and five distinct pIs from the 20 kDa molecules from all the T cell clones tested, both T4+ and T8+, thereby confirming their invariant nature. By comparison, the 43 kDa molecules co-precipitated by anti-CD3 showed considerable variability by pI analysis, suggesting peptide heterogeneity. Peptide maps confirmed this heterogeneity of the 43 kDa β-chain molecules from several clones, and in addition, some variability of the 49 kDa α-chain molecules was suggested, consistent with the view that these chains could participate in antigen recognition.

The Reinherz group then reasoned that if the clone-specific MoAbs actually recognized the antigen-binding chains of the TCR, they might also mimic antigen, and activate the T cell clones, provided they were presented on a solid support.[5] Thus, individual clone-specific MoAbs were conjugated to Sepharose beads. As controls, anti-T3, anti-T4 and anti-T8 MoAbs were also conjugated to

Sepharose. When tested for their capacity to induce IL-2 production and proliferation as monitored by ^{3}H-TdR, the results were clear-cut. Only anti-T3 and the appropriate anti-Ti induced both IL-2 production and proliferation of both T4 and T8 cytolytic clones. Moreover, only soluble anti-T3 and the appropriate anti-Ti were capable of inhibiting IL-2 production and proliferation induced by the solid-phase MoAbs. Subsequently, they repeated these experiments using helper/inducer T4$^+$ clones specific for soluble protein antigens, with identical results.[3] As concluded by the Reinherz team, "*these results provide compelling evidence to support the notion that anti-Ti antibodies define the antigen* (recognition) *receptor structure on individual clones.*"

They also pointed out that the T4 and T8 surface structures, although critical for MHC-restricted CTL effector function, were unnecessary for solid-phase MoAb-induced IL-2 production and clonal proliferation. Their results also indicated that endogenous IL-2 production was inseparable from clonal proliferation, and it was clear that a single cell could, under physiological conditions, both produce and respond to its own IL-2. Accordingly, the molecules involved in antigen recognition and response in adaptive immunity were thus resolved and revealed.

Additional experiments focused on the biochemical characterization of the α-chains and β-chains reactive with the clone-specific MoAbs showed that the α subunits were more acidic than the b subunits by IEF, and more importantly, two-dimensional peptide maps indicated that the β-chains precipitated from two distinct clones were unique, but did share two peptides in common.[6] By comparison, a similar analysis of α subunits from different clones were more related, but not identical. Therefore, both subunits appeared to contain both constant and variable domains, similar to antibodies.

Accordingly, these initial molecular characterizations indicated some similarities between the αβ antigen recognition elements of the TCR and antibodies. However, there the similarities ended, in that an invariant component like T3 involved in signaling had not been found to be associated with surface immunoglobulin on B cells. Also, B cells did not express accessory molecules similar to T4 and T8 as did T cells. Moreover, the data accumulated by Reinherz's group indicated that restriction of T cell antigen recognition to MHC class I or class II correlated with the expression of T8 or T4, respectively. It was also noteworthy that the T8/class I and T4/class II interaction did not necessarily dictate T cell function of cytolysis vs. help, since T4/class II-restricted T cell clones could obviously kill appropriate target cells. Finally, these data indicated that only one 90 kDa heterodimeric TCR antigen receptor could recognize alloantigens, and only one receptor could recognize foreign protein antigens, such as ragweed extract E and Tetanus Toxoid + MHC encoded molecules simultaneously. All of these findings were summarized in January, 1983.[7]

Confirmatory Data

A few months before Reinherz's first report on the molecular nature of the entire TCR complex,[1] James Allison and his students reported in 1982 that they had generated a MoAb reactive with a surface antigen of a T cell lymphoma. Their data indicated that *"the MoAb was highly specific for the T lymphoma cells used for the immunizations, and did not react with a panel of other spontaneous or X-ray-induced or chemically-induced lymphomas."*[8] Of interest, on biochemical analysis of surface radiolabeled proteins, the MoAb precipitated *"a glycoprotein composed of disulfide bonded subunits of 39,000 and 41,000 m.w."* In addition, Allison's group used a technique of "diagonal" two-dimensional gel electrophoresis combining an SDS-PAGE under non-reducing conditions followed by re-electrophoresis under reducing conditions. Because most surface molecules are not disulfide linked, most of the proteins migrated on a diagonal under these conditions. However, the disulfide linked proteins reactive with the MoAb migrated off the diagonal, because when reduced, the two chains separated into their lower sizes.

Operating under the hypothesis that the lymphoma-specific antigen recognized by their MoAb might be part of a surface molecule normally expressed specifically by T cells, the Allison group subjected several different types of cells to two-dimensional non-reducing/reducing SDS-PAGE. They found that purified T cells and thymocytes had proteins migrating off the diagonal in positions very similar to the MoAb immunoprecipitated proteins from the T cell lymphoma. By comparison, bone marrow cells (mostly myeloid and erythroid precursors) and B cells did not express detectable proteins migrating in this manner. The Allison team speculated that their MoAb might recognize the "*T cell equivalent of the B cell idiotype*," but because they had raised their MoAb against a tumor cell, they had no way to test for antigen recognition or immunological reactivity, in contrast to Reinherz, who had used normal functional IL-2-dependent T cell clones.

Then, a few months after Reinherz's first seminal report, another group led by Philippa Marrack reported in 1983 the generation of a MoAb reactive with an antigen-specific murine somatic T cell hybrid that they had produced by fusing immune Balb/c splenocytes with an azaguanine-resistant thymoma cell line.[9] This "T cell hybridoma," DO-11.10, was selected for its capacity to produce IL-2 when stimulated with specific antigen, chicken ovalbumin (cOVA), in the presence of APCs of the appropriate MHC type. Then, splenocytes from a DO-11.10-immunized mouse were used to make a B cell hybridoma, which was screened for the capacity to inhibit the production of IL-2 by cOVA-stimulated T cell hybrids. Supernatants from one cloned hybridoma, KJ1-26, was selected for study. The KJ1-26 MoAb-containing supernatants selectively inhibited IL-2 production only from the immunizing T cell hybridoma, and not from six other antigen-specific T cell hybridomas. In addition, this MoAb specifically inhibited binding of the DO-11.10 hybridoma to antigen-pulsed APCs, suggesting that the KJ1-26 MoAb might recognize a surface structure that bound antigen.

Identification of the molecules reactive with the KJ1-26 MoAb revealed that it immunoprecipitated a molecule of ~80–90 kDa by SDS-PAGE under non-reducing conditions and two molecules of 40–44 kDa under reducing conditions. Like the Allison group's experiments using "diagonal" non-reducing/reducing SDS-PAGE, the KJ1-26 immunoprecipitates revealed a spot that was below the diagonal, consistent with its disulfide-bonded structure. Accordingly, like the Allison group, the Marrack group had generated a MoAb that reacted with an antigen of similar biochemical characteristics expressed by a T cell hybridoma, and in addition, they had data showing that the MoAb blocked antigen-specific MHC-restricted IL-2 production. However, neither the Allison nor the Marrack groups had data revealing any other T cell functions such as proliferation or cytolysis, as they were dealing with hybridoma cells that proliferated autonomously. Also, there were no data regarding the T3 signaling components of the TCR complex, nor the nature of the MHC restricting structures T4 and T8. Their reports on the biochemical characteristics of the putative antigen recognition elements in these mouse lymphoma cells and hybridoma cells thus confirmed Reinherz's findings regarding the antigen recognition elements of the human TCR complex, but they did not describe the entire murine TCR complex on both T4-class II restricted and T8-class I-restricted T cell clones of both cytolytic as well as inducer/helper functional phenotypes, as had Reinherz's reports.

Once the data from all three groups became known to one another, they cooperated in their next reports, which were published simultaneously in the same journal. The Reinherz group reported the generation of an additional MoAb reactive with a human T cell leukemia/lymphoma cell line, which was T3+, T4+ and T8+.[10] Three MoAbs that reacted specifically only with this T cell tumor were selected for study. These MoAbs resembled the clone-specific MoAbs raised against the normal T cell clones, in that they did not react with normal T cells, B cells, macrophages, granulocytes or RBCs. Moreover, each of these tumor-specific MoAbs co-modulated clone-specific surface structures, as well as T3, but did not change the surface expression of T4, T8 or T11. SDS-PAGE analysis of immunoprecipitates under non-reducing conditions revealed a single band at 94 kDa, and two bands under reducing conditions (53 and 44 kDa). Peptide maps of the putative α and β chains showed that they were distinct molecules, and that they both shared peptide fragments in common with chains immunoprecipitated from normal T cell clones, thereby indicating that all of the clonotypic MoAbs precipitated chains that shared at least one peptide fragment, presumed constant domains, as well as clone-specific peptides, presumed variable domains. Also, using "diagonal" two-dimensional SDS-PAGE, the Reinherz group substantiated their earlier reports regarding the T cell phenotype during thymic maturation[11,12] by showing that the clone-specific TCR recognition molecules appear during intrathymic ontogeny in parallel with surface T3 expression, so that cells pass from triple negative (T3-T4-T8-) to double positive (T3-T4$^+$T8$^+$), to T3/Ti$^+$ and single positive for either T4 or T8. Thus, the clonotypic antigen recognition elements are intimately linked to T3 expression during ontogeny, thereby providing a structural basis for the group's previously reported observation that immunological competence is acquired only among the population of thymocytes that express surface T3 (13). In this regard, it is noteworthy that only this very minor subset of thymocytes (<10%), which also are cortisone resistant, were found responsive to LAF (IL-1), and thus capable of inducing proliferation in the LAF (IL-1) thymocyte bioassay because they could produce TCGF (IL-2).

The Marrack group reported data on a second MoAb, this one reactive with a T cell hybridoma that produced IL-2 in response to a class I alloantigen,[14] their first MoAb being specific for a T cell hybrid reactive with an MHC class II restricted cOVA antigen. This new MoAb, designated KJ12-98, suppressed IL-2 production by the class I-stimulated T cell hybrid, and in addition, when bound to Sepharose beads, stimulated IL-2 production, as Reinherz had shown for his clone-specific MoAbs. Also, like all the previous reports this MoAb precipitated a disulfide linked heterodimer, ~85 kDa, which resolved into two subunits of 40–43 kDa. Subsequently, Lawrence Samuelson and co-workers reported two MoAbs reactive with a class II-restricted T cell hybridoma that responded to a pigeon cytochrome C peptide by producing IL-2.[15] Like the MoAbs of the Marrack group, these MoAbs inhibited clone-specific antigen-induced IL-2 production, and precipitated disulfide-linked dimers comprising 45–50 kDa molecules.

By comparison, Bradley McIntyre and Allison used their MoAb to isolate the reactive antigen from their T cell lymphoma cell line, which they then used to immunize a rabbit to generate a polyclonal antiserum.[16] This antiserum precipitated disulfide-linked dimers from both normal thymocytes and peripheral T cells, but not non-T cells. Peptide maps indicated that the molecules from the different cell sources shared common subunits, as well as having non-homologous peptide fragments. However, they still did not have data indicating that either their MoAb or their antiserum reacted with a structure capable of recognizing antigens.

Accordingly, by the close of 1983 the enigmatic TCR complex had been revealed to all in the immunological community. From the chronology of the reports that appeared during this year, it is clear that the Reinherz group was first, complete and correct, as time would prove. By comparison, those working in the mouse necessarily followed Reinherz's lead, thereby partially confirming his findings, but because they lacked identification of murine T3 and T4, they could not describe all of the molecules of the entire TCR complex, and consequently they could not trace the expression of the recognition, accessory, or signaling elements during T cell ontogeny as did Reinherz. Moreover, because they chose to work with continuously proliferating T cell lymphomas and hybridomas instead of using normal IL-2-dependent T cell clones, they could not examine the function of the TCR complex in T cell activation, proliferation and any differentiated function such as cytolysis, beyond showing that their MoAbs interfered with antigen-induced IL-2 production.

cDNA Clones Encoding T Cell-Specific Membrane Proteins

All the data accumulated by Reinherz on the molecular nature of the TCR complex indicated that human T cells expressed surface molecules distinct from B cells that were involved in antigen recognition, as well as the T3 signaling molecules and the T4 and T8 accessory molecules associated with MHC restriction. The data accumulated on the αβ antigen recognition chains indicated that they were of a different size compared with the heavy and light chains of antibodies, but like antibodies, the TCR chains did appear to have both constant and variable regions.

Thus, Tak Mak's group took these data into consideration in 1984 to search for the cDNAs encoding the TCR antigen recognition molecules.[17] They screened for cDNA clones of mRNAs that were expressed either exclusively or preferentially in T cells, in contrast with others who had searched for Ig molecules on both B cells and T cells.[18] Given the T cell-specific expression of T3, T4 and T8 as parts of the TCR complex, they constructed a cDNA library from mRNA extracted from the human leukemia cell line MOLT3, which they found to express T3, T4 and T8.[19] Of 10,000 cDNA clones screened by differential hybridization to mRNA from MOLT3 cells vs. a human B cell lymphoma, four were selected for further study, which were found to identify a single mRNA of 1.3 kb by Northern blot analysis from MOLT3 that was not detected in the B cell line. Of several human leukemia cell lines screened, only T cell leukemias were positive by RNA/DNA hybridization, as well as normal human thymocytes and peripheral T cells, together with a mouse T cell leukemia cell line.

To determine the size of the protein encoded by their cDNA, they used hybrid selection with mRNA from MOLT3 cells, followed by *in vitro* translation and analysis by SDS-PAGE, which yielded a single protein of ~30 kDa. The nucleotide sequence of one of the cDNA clones revealed a long open reading frame that predicted a 34,938-kDa protein, two possible sites for N-linked glycosylation, a hydrophobic leader sequence at the N-terminus, and a hydrophobic region near the C-terminus resembling a membrane anchor. In addition, the predicted protein resembled human and murine Ig light chains, especially in the relative locations of the cysteine residues, as well as extensive homology over the entire length of the Ig variable, joining and constant regions. These results were very tantalizing, but there was no way to test for antigen recognition or any other function because they were dealing with cDNA from lymphoma cells. Moreover, even if this represented the cDNA encoding an antigen recognition component of the TCR complex, it represented only one of the two chains. Thus, the Mak group could only conclude that, *"The nature and function of this protein are unkown; it may be similar to the known T cell-specific antigens* (T3, T4, T8), *or to the α- or β-subunits of the recently identified T-cell receptors."*[17]

Following this report in the same journal issue, Stephen Hedrick, Mark Davis and their co-workers reported their work on a presumptive murine TCR antigen recognition structure.[20] Also operating from a hypothesis that the T cell antigen recognition elements should be specifically expressed by T cells and not by B cells, this team crafted a strategy of constructing ^{32}P-labeled cDNAs of the membrane-bound polysomal RNA fraction of murine antigen-specific T cell hybridomas, previously described by Samelson and co-workers,[15] assuming that mRNAs encoding a membrane molecule would be found on membrane-bound polysomes. They then subtracted these cDNAs by an excess of RNAs from B cell polysomes, to render the radiolabeled cDNA probes T cell-specific. T cell cDNA homologous to B cell RNA was removed by fractionation on hydroxyapatite, which binds double-stranded nucleotides. The resulting B cell-subtracted ^{32}P-cDNA was used to probe a cDNA library constructed with mRNA from another B cell-subtracted T cell cDNA preparation. From 5,000 clones screened, 30 were selected and used for further study. Seven clones hybridized with mRNA considered large enough to code for a TCR recognition element. They next hypothesized that the TCR recognition elements should undergo genetic rearrangements to create the diversity of antigen recognition in a manner similar to Ig genes. Thus, they constructed probes from each of the seven clones and hybridized them in Southern blots with genomic DNA from liver cells from the mouse strains used and genomic DNA from the parent T cell lymphoma used to construct the T cell hybridomas, as well as genomic DNA from the antigen-specific T cell hybridoma. Only one clone of the seven was consistent with DNA rearrangements, which were found only in the T cell lymphoma and hybridomas.

The nucleotide sequence of their longest cDNA clone predicted a leader sequence of 19 residues, a 98-residue region with similarity to murine Ig variable regions, a 16-amino acid J region, followed by a constant-like region, also similar to murine Ig constant regions. The similarity in sequence between the predicted T cell cDNA and Ig was so pronounced that it was conjectured that it could conceivably explain the reported cross-reactivity of B cell anti-idiotypic antisera with T cells.[18] Finally, there was a predicted hydrophobic membrane-spanning region near the C-terminus. Thus, the authors concluded that *"it must almost certainly play a part in antigen recognition by T cells."* In support of this contention, they cited unpublished work which indicated that antisera raised against peptide fragments predicted by their cDNA clone significantly inhibited the antigen-dependent release of IL-2 by antigen-stimulated T cell hybridomas.[21]

Another way to approach the primary sequence of a TCR antigen recognition molecule was to purify the α and/or β chains and perform N-terminal amino acid sequence analysis. Thus, the Reinherz group chose to use their clone-specific MoAbs reactive with their REX T-leukemia cell line because they could grow the requisite number of cells more easily than their IL-2-dependent T cell clones. Lysates from 5×10^{10} cells were immunoaffinity purified using their clonotypic MoAb. Focusing on the smaller β chain (~41–44 kDa), 20–50 μg of protein could be obtained from ~5×10^{10} cells. N-terminal sequencing reproducibly yielded the first 12 residues, minus the 1st amino acid. Comparison of this sequence with other proteins in the data base yielded a weak homology with a human Ig λ V-region.

The 1984 Reinherz report[22] was submitted for publication just three days before the cDNA sequences were reported. Thus, Reinherz added a note in the galley proof:

> *"Additional NH$_2$-terminal sequencing of Ti β subunit has identified amino acid residues 12, 14, and 16–20 and thus yields the following sequence: X-Val-Ile-Gln-Ser-Pro-Arg-His-Glu-Val-Thr-Glu-X-Gly-X-Glu-Val-Thr-Leu-Arg. These 17 amino acids are identical to 17 residues within the predicted protein sequence of the YT35 cDNA clone defined by Yanagi et al. (1984) ... In addition, the high degree of nucleotide homology between the 3'-end of the YT35 human cDNA clone and murine cDNA clones[21] ... suggests that the mouse equivalent of the Ti β gene has (also) been isolated."[22]*

Thus, by two different methods, protein and nucleotide sequencing, the primary structure of the first TCR complex antigen recognition chain became known. In addition, the two methods validated each other.

Turning Antigen-specific Activation into Antigen-nonspecific Action

From all these data, it appeared that although triggering of the TCR complex initiates T cell proliferative clonal expansion, there was a heretofore-unknown molecular mechanism that actually mediated the complex intracellular biochemical reactions that perform the necessary molecular events that culminate in DNA replication and cytokinesis. In this regard, one of the puzzling aspects of T cell proliferation after mitogenic or antigenic stimulation was the transient nature of the proliferative response. As noted by Peter Nowell in 1960, after the addition of a mitogenic lectin such as PHA, there ensues an initial lag of 48–72 hours, then a rapid burst of proliferation, followed by a gradual cessation of proliferative activity and ultimately a cessation of proliferation.[23] Once it was appreciated that the TCR complex is responsible for IL-2 production, and as well, once it became possible to monitor the TCR complex induction of IL-2R expression, these critical parameters regulating the T cell proliferative response could be examined. It appeared that the TCR complex *per se* could not promote DNA replication and cytokinesis.

From our initial 1978 studies of IL-2 production after mitogenic lectin triggering, we already knew that there was a burst of IL-2 secretion by the activated cells, followed by a gradual cessation of IL-2 release, and the disappearance of detectable IL-2 concentrations over the succeeding several days.[24] Therefore, this phenomenon alone could explain the transience of the proliferative response. However, once it became possible to monitor IL-2R expression, both quantitatively with the radiolabeled IL-2 binding assay, and qualitatively by flow cytometry using the IL-2R MoAb, in 1983 Doreen Cantrell performed a series of experiments on the biological importance of IL-2R expression.[25] Using IL-2 rendered homogeneous by MoAb immunoaffinity purification, biosynthetically radiolabeled IL-2 also immunoaffinity purified with the IL-2-reactive MoAbs, and IL-2R-reactive MoAbs, the growth characteristics of PHA-activated T cells were determined and correlated with IL-2R expression for the first time. IL-2Rs appear asynchronously in lectin-activated human peripheral T cell populations and *precede* the onset of DNA synthesis monitored by ^{3}H-TdR incorporation, as well as by propidium iodide (PI) quantitative DNA staining and flow cytometry. Moreover, upon removal of the activating lectin at the peak of IL-2R expression after 72 hours of culture, IL-2R levels do not persist. Rather, a time-related and IL-2 independent decay of IL-2Rs occurs that is rapidly reversible by re-stimulation with lectin. As IL-2R appearance and disappearance is mirrored and followed by the proliferative rate of the cells within the population, our results indicated that the lectin-induced IL-2R densities were of primary importance, along with adequate IL-2 concentrations, in determining the extent of T cell clonal expansion, and consequently by extrapolation, the tempo, magnitude and duration of the resultant T cell immune response.[25]

Although these studies were definitive about IL-2 and IL-2Rs, because we had performed the experiments using a mitogenic lectin as the activating signal, we could not be sure whether they represented the true physiology of the adaptive T cell immune response. Thus, it was a natural extension of these studies for us to collaborate with Ellis Reinherz's group, once he had established normal human T cell clones, and had generated clone-specific MoAbs. Accordingly, combining Reinherz's unique cellular and molecular TCR complex reagents with our unique IL-2 and IL-2R molecular reagents, for the first time it was possible to perform reductionist science on the molecular nature of the T cell adaptive immune response, thereby moving from the micrometer to the nanometer level in immunology in 1984.[26]

To investigate the relationship between the TCR complex and IL-2-mediated T cell growth, we used three antigen-specific human T cell clones and a series of clone-specific MoAbs in conjunction with homogeneous immunoaffinity-purified human IL-2, as well as MoAbs reactive with both IL-2 and the IL-2R. First, we established that two human cytolytic T cell clones (T4$^+$ and T8$^+$), and a protein antigen-specific helper/inducer T4$^+$ clone, proliferated *in vitro* in response to homogeneous purified IL-2, thus consistent with our studies that the active ingredient in LyCM was IL-2. Second, this IL-2-dependent proliferative response was essentially completely abrogated by the IL-2R MoAb, and was reduced from 67%–75% by the neutralizing IL-2-reactive MoAb. In contrast, MoAbs reactive with the constant portion of the human Ia antigen (MHC class II), that like the IL-2R appears on activated human T cells, did not diminish IL-2-mediated clonal proliferation.[26]

As observed previously with LyCM containing IL-2, we found that activation using soluble clone-specific MoAbs enhanced by 2–3-fold ^{3}H-TdR incorporation of each clone in response to pure homogeneous IL-2. As with IL-2 alone, this increased ^{3}H-TdR incorporation initiated by the anti-clonotype MoAbs was completely abrogated by the IL-2R-reactive MoAb and reduced by 2/3 by the MoAb that could neutralize IL-2. Since anti-clonotypic MoAbs did not promote proliferation without exogenous IL-2, we surmised that the soluble MoAbs may trigger the expression of IL-2Rs but not IL-2 production. This hypothesis was tested by flow cytometry. The expression of IL-2Rs was found to be stimulated 6-fold by stimulation with anti-clonotypic MoAb, and as well, by specific antigen + APCs. Accordingly, these data confirmed and extended our previous results using PHA, to the physiologic reagents of anti-clonotypic MoAb, and specific Ag + APCs.

Further experiments comparing activation with soluble vs. solid-phase anti-clonotypic MoAbs, and either cellular alloantigens or Ag + APCs, showed that soluble anti-clonotypic MoAbs promoted IL-2R expression but not IL-2 production, whereas the same anti-clonotypic MoAbs bound to Sepharose beads promoted both the expression of IL-2Rs and IL-2 production, as did both alloantigens and Ag + APCs. Thus, "*The present construct clearly implies that T cell proliferation is mediated through an autocrine network in which antigen-receptor triggering leads to IL-2 production, IL-2R expression, IL-2 release, and subsequent IL-2R occupancy, which ultimately promotes cell division.*"[26]

During these experiments, we noted that IL-2R expression after TCR complex activation occurred asynchronously among the individual cells within a T cell population. Moreover, examination at the single cell level using the cytofluorograph and IL-2R MoAbs, a broad range of IL-2Rs/cell was observed, spanning as much as three orders of magnitude. Accordingly, we wondered whether differences in IL-2R density made any difference to the IL-2-dependent proliferative response. In this regard, a purview of the literature revealed that all cells, both prokaryotes and eukaryotes, proliferate asynchronously, with some cells proliferating faster than others, even among cloned cell populations. Thus, we wondered whether this universal characteristic pattern of cell growth could be related to the density of growth factor receptors as well as the concentration of the growth factor.

Thus in 1984, for the first time in any cell system, we had accumulated the necessary molecular and cellular reagents to explore this fundamental aspect of cellular proliferation. Of utmost importance, a T cell population could be synchronized into the G_0-G_1 phase of the cell cycle by removal of IL-2, and then maximal levels of IL-2Rs could be induced by re-stimulation with mitogenic lectins. Upon exposure to IL-2, the kinetics of IL-2-dependent cell cycle progression could then be followed and analyzed in relationship to IL-2R density and distribution among the cells within the population.[27]

When the density of IL-2Rs is monitored by the cytofluorograph with IL-2R MoAbs, and plotted on a log_{10} scale, like all surface molecules, a log-normal distribution of IL-2Rs is observed. Since the proportion of occupied receptors is dependent on the IL-2 concentration, with a log-normal distribution of IL2Rs/cell, at any given IL-2 concentration the absolute number of occupied IL-2Rs should vary according to the receptor density of each cell. It follows that if the number of occupied IL-2Rs is critical for the decision to replicate DNA, a G_0-G_1 synchronized cell population with a log-normal distribution of IL-2Rs would be expected to enter the proliferative phases of the cell cycle asynchronously, as a function of the IL-2 concentration, which was readily observed. The IL-2 concentration-dependency was most easily discerned by selecting a single time interval after addition of IL-2: a typical sigmoid log-dose response curve resulted whether the response was monitored by ^{3}H-TdR incorporation or PI staining, which indicated that the magnitude of ^{3}H-TdR incorporation reflected the proportion of cells that had left G_0-G_1 and entered the proliferative phases of the cell cycle.[27]

In other experiments, the duration of the IL-2/IL-2R interaction was found to be a critical determinant of cell cycle progression, so that there appeared to be an interplay between at least two variables, IL-2 concentration and the duration of the IL-2/IL-2R interaction, such that the number of cells responsive to a suboptimal IL-2 concentration could be increased by lengthening the exposure period. These observations suggested that the absolute number of IL-2/IL-2R interactions occurring during the G_1 phase of the cell cycle was critical for the decision of a cell to divide. A series of experiments varying the IL-2 concentration, the IL-2R density or the duration that these two molecules interacted proved this hypothesis, and for the first time showed that cellular division is a deterministic and not a probabilistic phenomenon. Moreover, the decision is quite simple and depends upon only four variables: (1) the affinity of the IL-2/IL-2 interaction, which dictates (2) the IL-2 concentrations necessary to saturate the IL-2Rs, but (3) the IL-2R density/cell, and (4) the duration of the IL-2/IL-2R interaction are equally important.[27]

In just five years, the understanding of adaptive immunity underwent a sea-change, from a science focused on populations of cells to one focused on individual cells and molecules for the first time. No longer was the T cell antigen receptor complex, both structurally and functionally, an enigma. Gone were the notions that T cells recognized antigens via Ig molecules, although the antigen recognition structures were found to be members of what came to be known as the Ig superfamily. Moreover, the TCR complex became defined as comprising of antigen recognition structures of α- and β-chains, as well as accessory molecules, T4 and T8, that facilitated recognition of antigens "in the context" of MHC-encoded molecules, and which were found to be intimately involved in T cell ontogeny. Moreover, the TCR complex included the T3 signaling molecules, which were expressed by all T cells. Also gone were antigen-specific factors, as T cells were not found to secrete their antigen-recognition structures, as do B cells. Moreover, the MHC-encoded molecules also were shown not to be TCRs, and not to be secreted as helper or suppressor 'factors.' Rather, the genetic control of the T cell immune response was found to be involved with antigen presentation via

MHC-encoded molecules, which T cells recognize via only one receptor, not two. In addition, T cells were found to mediate their antigen-specific responses via signaling the expression of antigen non-specific molecules, the cytokines or interleukins, and their receptors. Consequently, the immune response could no longer be considered a unique, passive system that only functioned in response to external signals from the environment. Like all the other bodily systems, the immune system became appreciated for the first time to be regulated by endogenous hormone-like molecules via specific hormone-like receptors. These changes in our perception of how the adaptive immune system is structured and how it functions led immediately to a new vista of experimental and therapeutic possibilities, one where the exploration of a myriad of new molecules and biochemical signaling pathways have made immunology one of the most interesting and rapidly expanding areas of biology, and one where it is now on its way to contribute in a major way to 21st century medicine. Moreover, to launch this quest, the torch was passed to a new generation of immunologists armed with cloned genes, cloned cells, cloned antibodies and cloned cytokines, reagents that were transformative for the new science of molecular immunology.

References

1. Meuer SC, Fitzgerald KA, Hussey RE, Hodgdon JC, Schlossman S and Reinherz EL. (1983). Clonotypic structures involved in antigen-specific human T cell function. Relationship to the T3 molecular comlex. *J Exp Med* **157**:705–719.
2. Meuer S, Acuto O, Hussey R, Hodgdon J, Fitzgerald K, Schlossman S and Reinherz E. (1983). Evidence for the T3-associated 90K heterodimer as the T cell antigen receptor. *Nature* **303**:808–810.
3. Meuer S, Cooper D, Hodgdon J, Hussey R, Fitzgerald K, Schlossman S and Reinherz E. (1983). Identification of the receptor for antigen and major histocompatability complex on human inducer T lymphocytes. *Science* **222**:1239–1242.
4. Reinherz E, Meuer S, Fitzgerald K, Hussey R, Hodgdon J, Acuto O and Schlossman S. (1983). Comparison of T3-associated 49- and 43-kilodalton cell surface molecules on individual human T cell clones: Evidence for

peptide variability in T-cell receptor structures. *Proc Natl Acad Sci USA* **80**:4104–4108.

5. Meuer SC, Hodgdon JC, Hussey RE, Protentis JP, Schlossman S and Reinherz EL. (1983). Antigen-like effects of monoclonal antibodies directed at receptors on human T cell clones. *J Exp Med* **158**:988–993.

6. Acuto O, Meuer S, Hodgdon J, Schlossman S and Reinherz E. (1983). Peptide variability exists within alpha and beta subunits of the T cell receptor for antigen. *J Exp Med* **158**:1368–1373.

7. Reinherz E, Meuer S and Sclossman S. (1983). The delineation of antigen receptors on human T lymphocytes. *Immunology Today* **4**:5–8.

8. Allison J, McIntyre B and Bloch D. (1982). Tumor-specific antigen of murine T-lymphoma defined with monoclonal antibody. *J Immunol* **129**: 2293–2300.

9. Haskins K, Kubo R, Pigeon M, White J, Kappler J and Marrack P. (1983). The major histocompatability compex restricted antigen receptor in T cells. I. Isolation with a monoclonal antibody. *J Exp Med* **157**:1149–1158.

10. Acuto O, Hussey R, Fitzgerald K, Protentis J, Meuer S, Schlossman S and Reinherz E. (1983). The human T cell receptor: Appearance in ontogoney and biochemical relationship of alpha and beta subunits on IL2-dependent clones and T cell tumors. *Cell* **34**:717–726.

11. Reinherz E, Kung P, Goldstein G, Levey R and Schlossman S. (1980). Discrete stages of intrathymic differentiation: Analysis of normal thymocytes and leukemic lymphoblasts of T cell lineage. *Proc Natl Acad Sci USA* **77**:1588–1592.

12. Reinherz EL and Schlossman SF. (1980). The differentiation and function of T lymphocytes. *Cell* **4**:821–827.

13. Umiel T, Daley J, Bahn A, Levey R, Schlossman S and Reinherz E. (1982). Acquisition of immune competence by a subset of human cortical thymocytes expressing mature T cell antigens. *J Immunol* **129**:1054–1060.

14. Kappler J, Kubo R, Haskins K, White J and Marrack P. (1983). The mouse T cell receptor: Comparison of MHC-restricted receptors on two T cell hybridomas. *Cell* **34**:727–737.

15. Samelson L, Germain R and Schwartz R. (1983). Monoclonal antibodies against the antigen receptor on a cloned T cell hybrid. *Proc Natl Acad Sci USA* **80**:6972–6976.

16. McIntyre B and Allison J. (1983). The mouse T cell receptor: Structural heterogeneity of molecules of normal T cells defined by xenoantiserum. *Cell* **34**: p739–746.

17. Yanagi Y, Yoshikai Y, Leggett K, Clark S, Aleksander I and Mak T. (1984). A human T cell-specific cDNA clone encodes a protein having extensive homology to immunoglobulin chains. *Nature* **308**:145–149.

18. Binz H and Wigzell H. (1975). Shared idiotypic determinants on B and T lymphocytes reactive against the same antigenic determinants. I. Demonstration of similar or identical idiotypes on IgG molecules and T-cell receptors with specificity for the same alloantigens. *J Exp Med* **142**:197–211.

19. Nagasawa K and Mak TW. (1982). Induction of differentiation in human T-lymphoblastic leukemia cell lines by 12-O-tetradecanoylphorbol 13-acetate (TPA): Studies with monoclonal antibodies to T cells. *Cellular immunology* **71**:396–403.

20. Hedrick S, Cohen D, Nielson E and Davis MM. (1984). Isolation of cDNA clones encoding T cell-specific membrane associated proteins. *Nature* **308**:149–155.

21. Hedrick S, Nielson E, Kavaler J, Cohen D and Davis M. (1984). Sequence relationships between putative T cell receptor polypeptides and immunoglobulins. *Nature* **308**:153–158.

22. Acuto O, Fabbi M, Smart J, Poole C, Protentis J, Royer H, Schlossman S and Reinherz E. (1984). Purification and NH2-terminal amino acid sequencing of the beta subunit of a human T-cell antigen receptor. *Proc Natl Acad Sci USA* **81**:3851–3855.

23. Nowell PC. (1960). Phytohemagglutinin: An initiator of mitosis in cultures of normal human leukocytes. *Cancer Research* **20**:462–468.

24. Gillis S, Ferm MM, Ou W and Smith KA. (1978). T cell growth factor: Parameters of production and a quantitative microassay for activity. *J Immunol* **120**:2027–2032.

25. Cantrell, D.A. and Smith, K.A. (1983). Transient expression of interleukin 2 receptors. Consequences for T cell growth. *J Exp Med* **158**:1895–1911.

26. Meuer SC, Hussey RE, Cantrell DA, Hodgen JC, Schlossman SF, Smith KA and Reinherz EL. (1984). Triggering the T3-Ti antigen-receptor complex results in clonal T cell proliferation through an interleukin 2-dependent autocrine pathway. *PNAS* **81**:1509–1513.

27. Cantrell DA and Smith KA. (1984). The interleukin-2 T-cell system: A new cell growth model. *Science* **224**:1312–1316.

4. Molecular Mechanisms of T Cell Cytolysis

TCR Signals

From the days of Nowell, T cell "activation" was synonymous with mitogen/antigen stimulation that resulted in T cell proliferation.[1] Indeed, because tritiated thymidine (^{3}H-TdR) incorporation was generally used as the read-out for T cell activation, it was assumed by everyone that the trigger for T cell proliferation resided solely with activation of the T cell antigen receptor complex. However, with the realization that there is a molecular mechanism whereby TCR/CD3 signaling initiates proliferation, comprising an endogenous hormone that triggers a hormone-like receptor, it became possible for the first time to begin to separate the biochemical signals generated by triggering the TCR from those triggered by the interleukin-2 receptor (IL-2R).

Carol Deutsch first provided evidence in 1979 that an early event in mitogenic triggering of lymphocytes might involve changes in the intracellular concentration and/or transport of cations (e.g. potassium, calcium).[2] Since the transmembrane electrical potential is an important factor in the movement of charged ions across the plasma membrane, Deutsch carefully measured it in human peripheral blood mononuclear cells (PBMCs), and found it to be between −35 mV and −52 mV. These results implied that ion gradients are maintained by energy-dependent processes in these cells, which were not generally considered excitable cells, like neurons.

Subsequently, in 1982 Roger Tsien took advantage of the newly available calcium-specific fluorescent indicator, Quin2, which made possible the first direct measurements of intracellular [Ca^{2+}] in mouse thymocytes and pig lymph node cells using a spectrofluorometer.[3] Mitogenic lectins such as phytohemagglutinin (PHA), Concanavalin-A (Con-A) and calcium ionophores (A23187, ionomycin) raised intracellular calcium concentration within a few minutes. Of note, deprivation of extracellular calcium prevented the response. Moreover, the lectin-induced intracellular [Ca^{2+}] increases were sufficient to hyperpolarize the membrane potential, from −50 mV to −70 mV, which the authors speculated was likely due to a K$^+$ conductance.

Yasutomi Nishizuka provided insight regarding the biochemical mechanism(s) whereby various cell surface receptors could transfer informational signals from the cell surface into the cellular interior with his early 1980s pathbreaking reports of two routes, protein kinase-C (PKC) activation and Ca^{2+} mobilization.[4,5] The signal-dependent breakdown of inositol phospholipids, particularly phophotidylinositol bisphosphate (PIP$_2$), was found to be the key event for initiating these processes. After stimulation of surface receptors, PIP$_2$ is degraded immediately to produce 1,2-diacylglycerol and inositol 1,4,5-triphosphate (IP$_3$). He showed that this turnover of membrane phospholipids is associated with an increase in intracellular [Ca^{2+}], and the diacylglcerol produced initiates the activation of a calcium-dependent protein kinase (PKC). Thus, the extracellular receptor triggering information is transferred directly across the lipid membrane bilayer via the breakdown of membrane phospholipids and ultimately results in intracellular protein phosphorylation.

Although these reports were suggestive that perhaps TCR/CD3 triggering could very well operate via this newly discovered transmembrane signaling mechanism, the step from polyclonal mitogenic activation vs. monoclonal activation remained to be defined. Accordingly, in 1984 Ellis Reinherz and collaborators used flow cytometry to analyze Quin2 fluorescence upon anti-TCR MoAb as well as anti-CD3 MoAb activation of T cell clones.[6] When coupled to Sepharose beads, anti-TCR and anti-CD3 both caused a rapid increase in intracellular [Ca^{2+}]. It is noteworthy that IL-2 did not cause any change in intracellular [Ca^{2+}], despite promoting cellular proliferation. Also, removal of extracellular calcium using the chelator EGTA blocked anti-TCR and anti-CD3-induced proliferation of both cytolytic and helper/inducer T cell clones, but particularly noteworthy, did not prevent IL-2-mediated proliferation.

Others took advantage of the human T cell leukemic cell line, JURKAT, which had been found to produce IL-2 when stimulated with mitogenic lectins.[7,8] Also in 1984 Arthur Weiss, working in John Stobo's group showed that JURKAT clones would also produce IL-2 when activated by soluble anti-CD3, provided phorbol myristic acetate (PMA), which Nishizuka had shown to activate PKC, was also present.[9] Weiss and coworkers then showed that soluble anti-CD3 MoAbs promoted a rapid increase in intracellular $[Ca^{2+}]$, as did PHA and calcium ionophore, and that the combination of PMA + Ionophore promoted the production of IL-2.[10] Accordingly, these studies indicated that activation of both PKC and a rapid increase in intracellular $[Ca^{2+}]$ were required to promote IL-2 production, and taken together with Reinherz's results, they indicated that solid phase but not soluble MoAbs reactive with either the antigen recognition chains of clone-specific TCRs or the pan-T cell signaling complex, CD3, activated both PKC and an increase in intracellular $[Ca^{2+}]$. By comparison, IL-2 did not appear to operate via this pathway. Moreover, exactly what transpired between these early biochemical changes in T cells, which occurred within minutes of TCR/CD3 triggering, and the activation of IL-2 gene expression, which required at least an hour of continuous TCR/CD3 stimulation remained to be explored.

Molecular Mechanisms of Cell-mediated Cytolysis (CMC)

Subsequent to the original 1968 description of cell-mediated lysis of ^{51}Cr-labeled target cells,[11] the mechanisms responsible for this phenomenon remained obscure, especially at the molecular level. However, Pierre Henkart's team first showed in 1980 via electron microscopy that human mononuclear cells punctured tubular holes into the membranes of susceptible target cells during antibody-dependent cellular cytotoxicity (ADCC), very similar to the morphology of complement-mediated lysis.[12]

Subsequently, in 1983 Eckhard Podack and Gunther Dennert found that cloned murine natural killer (NK) cells[13] and cloned alloantigen-specific murine IL-2-dependent CTL[14] produced similar circular membrane lesions in target cells that arose by membrane insertion of tubular complexes, which they conjectured were assembled from subunits during the cytolytic reaction, like the terminal components of complement. The tubules were detected on target cell membranes by immune electron microscopy and appeared to form transmembrane channels as seen in ultrathin sections.

To move toward a molecular explanation of these observations, Podack was ideally situated because he had already studied the complement components for several years with Hans Muller-Eberhard. Even so, a major hurdle remained to be surmounted to move from these analytical morphological descriptions to a detailed molecular analysis of the phenomena. One of our perplexing findings noted as soon as we had successfully created the first Cytotoxic T Lymphocyte Lines (CTLL)[15] and clones[16] was the appearance of the CTLL upon light and electron microscopy. The cytoplasm of the cells after methanol fixation and procession for staining by Wright-Giemsa revealed many granule-shaped cytoplasmic holes. Electron microscopy revealed that these organelles contained electron dense material. Podack hypothesized that these putative granules were the elusive cytotoxic granules of CTL, so that he took advantage of the capacity to grow up large numbers of CTLL-2 in IL-2-containing Con-A T cell Supernatant (CATSUP). He generated $> 10^9$ cells that he used to isolate and purify the cytoplasmic granules. The plasma membranes were disrupted by N_2 cavitation, and post nuclear supernatants were applied to self-generated Percoll density gradients, fractions of which were analyzed by structural analysis using electron microscopy, and for function by assaying for cytolytic activity in the presence and absence of calcium using sheep and rabbit erythrocytes as targets. The fractions containing very pure granules by EM yielded detectable cytolytic activity.[17] SDS-PAGE of the fractions containing cytolytic activity revealed six characteristic bands, ranging in molecular sizes from 75 kDa to 10 kDa under reducing conditions. This 1984 study represented the first demonstration of strong, calcium-dependent cytolytic activity of isolated CTL granules. Similar results for cytolytic granules isolated from Large Granular Lymphocyte (LGL) tumor cells were reported by Pierre and Maryanna Henkart and their co-workers, so that it appeared that both CTL and NK cells lysed target cells using similar granules.[18]

One year later in 1985, to approach the purification of the active proteins found in the cytolytic granules, Podack together with John Young and Zanvil Cohen,[19] prepared 5 mL of packed cells from 6L cultures of CTLL-2 cells grown in 10%–15% CATSUP. Granules with cytolytic activity purified from these packed cells via Percoll density-gradient centrifugation were mixed with 1 M phosphate buffer (pH 7.4), which precipitated the Percoll, allowing its easy removal by centrifugation. The transparent supernatant was then purified via gel filtration, fractions from which were assayed for protein and hemolytic activity, then pooled and further purified via ion exchange High Pressure Liquid Chromatography (HPLC). Hemolytic fractions from this column were pooled and analyzed by SDS-PAGE, which yielded a single 75 kDa protein, which was provisionally designated protein-1 (P1). Analysis for hemolytic activity showed that lysis was Ca^{2+}-dependent, inhibited by Zn^{2+} ions and accompanied by polymerization to form membrane-associated tubular complexes that formed large transmembrane pores, which caused rapid membrane depolarization in the presence of Ca^{2+}. Daniele Masson and Jurg Tschopp, simultaneously purified a similar single protein from the cytolytic granules of another IL-2-dependent CTL line, terming this protein "perforin".[20]

These findings led to the inevitable comparison of P1/perforin with C9, the terminal lytic component of complement, and the conjecture that P1/perforin and C9 might have arisen from a common ancestral cytolytic protein that subsequently became specialized in cell-mediated and humoral cytolysis, respectively. To pursue this hypothesis, in 1986 Podack and his collaborators generated mono-specific antisera reactive to both denatured and native C9 and P1/perforin.[21] Cross-reactivity with P1/perforin and C9 was found using antisera reactive with denatured proteins but not by antisera reactive with native proteins, thereby indicating that the two proteins shared primary sequence epitopes, but not necessarily tertiary epitopes.

The next step, the identification and cloning of cDNA encoding P1/perforin, was accomplished by Podack's team in 1989 using the perforin-specific antisera and an expression λgt11 phage library constructed from murine CTLs.[22] The predicted amino acid sequence contained 554 residues and as expected, displayed considerable homology with certain functional domains of C9, C8α, C8β, and C7. Also noteworthy, consistent with Reinherz's finding of both CD8+ and CD4+ cytolytic T cell clones restricted to MHC class I and class II encoded molecules, perforin mRNA was detectable in both class I and class II restricted cytolytic T cell clones, but not in non-cytolytic T cell clones or in other non-cytolytic cells. Thus as predicted, in only a few years of the generation of monoclonal IL-2-dependent functional cytolytic T cells,[16] an initial molecular mechanism whereby cytolytic T cells kill target cells became evident for the first time.

In parallel, other investigators pursued a somewhat different path to discern the molecular mechanisms responsible for CMC. Tse Wen Chang and Herman Eisen reported in 1980 that an irreversible protease inhibitor, $N^{α}$-tosyl-L-lysyl-chloromethylketone (TLCK), markedly reduced MLC-generated CTL activity monitored by ^{51}Cr release assays.[23] Subsequently in 1984, Eisen's group demonstrated that murine alloreactive IL-2-dependent CTL clones had remarkably high serine esterase activity in detergent lysates.[24] By comparison, noncytolytic cells contained little, if any esterase activity. Of interest, cytolytic activity from CTL lysates, but not intact CTL activity, was inhibited completely by the irreversible esterase inhibitors, DFP and PMSF, suggesting that normally the serine esterase was located internally and not expressed on the cell surface.

Independently, a group led by Christopher Bleackley and another group led by Irving Weissman used CTL clones in 1986 to isolate and identify cDNA encoding novel T cell-specific serine proteases.[25–27] Then, a year later using the granules purified from two CTL clones, Masson and Tschopp isolated eight distinct serine proteases, designating them Granzymes A–H.[28] Accordingly, the prophecy that normal CTL clones and their granules would allow the identification of the molecular mechanisms of lymphocyte-mediated cytolysis proved prescient.[16] Even so, the identification of perforin/P1/cytolysin and Granzymes did not immediately answer the question as to how CTL and NK cells utilized these molecules to effect specific lysis of their target cells.

Apoptosis is a term from the Greek used to describe the "dropping off" or "falling off" of petals from flowers or leaves from trees. Kerr, Wyllie and Currie coined the term in 1972 to describe *"a general mechanism of controlled cell deletion, complimentary to mitosis in the regulation of cell populations"*.[29] They described cellular apoptosis as structural changes initiated or inhibited by a variety of environmental stimuli, involving nuclear and cytoplasmic condensation and breaking up of the cell into many membrane-bound, ultrastructurally well-preserved fragments.

John Russell and co-workers first showed in 1980 that CMC led to the release of both ^{51}Cr from the cytoplasm and $^{125}IUdR$ from the nucleus, whereas lysis of the same cells by antibody + complement or hypotonic shock led solely to the release of cytoplasmic ^{51}Cr.[30] Moreover, the intracellular disintegration of the nucleus occurred within minutes of CTL-target cell interaction, leading to two possible explanations, *"(1) The CTL injects degradative substances into the target cell, or (2) the target cell autolyzes itself in response to a signal from the CTL delivered at the plasma membrane"*.[31]

In 1983, Richard Duke and co-workers summarized the data accumulated on the mechanisms responsible for CMC, which could be separated into three distinguishable stages.[32] The first step involved target cell recognition and the establishment of a stable effector: target cell contact or conjugate. This step required Mg^{2+} or Ca^{2+}. The second step was found to be strictly Ca^{2+} dependent and constituted the "lethal hit" stage, during which the target cell was irreversibly committed to lysis. The third step involved effector cell independent target cell disintegration, wherein cytoplasmic macromolecules were released. Notably, all these steps were found to be independent of protein and RNA synthesis, which were known attributes of apoptosis in other cell systems. Nevertheless, operating with the hypothesis that CMC might entail an apoptotic mechanism, these investigators showed for the first time that within minutes of exposure of target cells to antigen-specific CTL, their nuclear DNA began to fragment and *preceded* cytoplasmic ^{51}Cr release by at least an hour. By comparison, killing mediated by heating, freeze/thawing or lysing with antibody and complement did not yield DNA fragmentation. Furthermore, agarose gel electrophoresis of target cell DNA showed discrete multiples of ~200 bp subunits, a characteristic of apoptosis, *"suggesting that DNA fragmentation was the result of activation of a specific endonuclease."*[32] Despite these findings, these investigators pointed out that CMC-mediated DNA fragmentation differed from other examples of apoptosis, in that it did not require transcription or translation, presumably necessary to produce an endogenous nuclease by the target cell.

One hypothesis that could serve to synthesize and reconcile all these experimental data, including the inhibition of CMC by specific protease inhibitors, was that the CTL granules contained a pore-forming protein, perforin/cytolysin, which provided the conduit through which granule proteases, granzymes, gained entrance to the target cell, liberating DNA, thereby leading to its rapid digestion. Accordingly, Pierre Henkart's group provided the first data in 1989 in support of this hypothesis: *"Although fully lytic concentrations of purified granule perforin/cytolysin alone failed to induce target cell DNA release, a combination of purified granzyme A and perforin/ cytolysin induces substantial DNA release."*[33] Subsequently in 1992, Arnold Greenberg's team reported similar findings from a serine esterase and cytolysin/perforin purified from a rat NK tumor cell line.[34] Consequently, two decades after the first description of ^{51}Cr release,[11] and a decade after the first description of cloned antigen-specific CTLs,[16] the molecular mechanisms responsible for CMC became evident to everyone.

Tolerance of Self via Negative Selection

In developing his Theory of Clonal Selection, Burnet necessarily had to account for the phenomenon of tolerance to self-bodily components that had been shown to develop during embryogenesis by Owen in 1945 and by Billingham, Brent and Medawar in 1953.[35,36]

Burnet stated:

"In the Burnet-Fenner theory (of antibody formation),[37] any potentialities of antibody production against body components were eliminated by the development of tolerance. In the present theory they are more readily disposed of by assuming that — at this particular stage of embryonic life — contact with the corresponding antigenic pattern results in the death of the cell. If the potential antigen persists long enough in high enough concentration, all clones which can produce this natural (auto) antibody will be eliminated."[38]

Of course, Burnet did not elaborate on the mechanism whereby self-reactive clones were eliminated, and this aspect of his theory had to be left to the future. Also, Burnet was writing before thymic-dependent maturation of T lymphocytes had been discovered,[39-41] so that his view of immunity was restricted to humoral immunity. Even so, by definition, tolerance had to be antigen-specific, because it resulted in the capacity of the immune system to ignore self-antigens specifically. Accordingly, Burnet had to propose that antigen-specific self-reactive clones must somehow be deleted or otherwise inactivated, i.e. rendered anergic, during embryogenesis.

Further progress in this area had to await the identification of surface immunoglobulin as the molecular basis of the B cell antigen receptor (BCR) in 1970,[42,43] and the elucidation of the molecular nature of the T cell antigen receptor (TCR), which required another decade.[44-46] Moreover, the generation of antibody-forming cells (AFC) to most antigens was inextricably linked to "help" derived from T cells, so that the underlying molecular basis for the development of B cell tolerance necessarily depended on understanding T cell tolerance.

A breakthrough in the search for the mechanism(s) underlying T cell tolerance was reported in 1987 by John Kappler and colleagues, who generated a monoclonal antibody (MoAb) that reacted with all T cells that expressed TCRs encoded by β-chain variable gene segments specified by the variable gene region Vβ17a.[47] Moreover, T cells bearing Vβ17a-encoded receptors that reacted with cells that expressed the major histocompatibility complex (MHC) class II protein, IE. Using this MoAb, it was found that T cells expressing Vβ17a were selectively eliminated from the mature thymocyte and peripheral T cell populations of mice expressing MHC class II IE, but were present in the expected numbers in immature thymocyte populations.[48] These observations were consistent with the notion, as proposed originally by Burnet, that tolerance to self-antigens (in this case self-MHC-encoded molecules) is due to clonal elimination. In addition, their findings indicated that the elimination of self-reactive thymocytes occurred in the thymus when immature thymocytes were selected to enter the mature thymocyte pool. All these experiments were possible because the Vβ17a TCRs amounted to as much as 10–20% of all the TCRs.

Despite these provocative findings, it remained unclear whether this phenomenon was restricted to recognition of MHC-encoded self-molecules, or indeed whether other so-called "nominal" self-antigens associated with MHC-encoded molecules would also react with particular TCR Vβ gene segments. Subsequently in 1988, while screening peripheral T cells and mature cortisone-resistant thymocytes from various inbred mouse strains using a MoAb that recognized all TCRs encoded by Vβ6 gene segments, Robson. MacDonald and co-workers made the serendipitous observation that Vβ6⁺ T cells correlated negatively with the expression of one allele of the 'minor lymphocyte–stimulating' (Mls) gene locus in all inbred mouse strains tested.[49] At the time of these studies, the structure and function of the Mls gene product(s) were unknown. However, Mls was remarkable, in that it was the only antigen other than the MHC-encoded molecules that could specifically stimulate proliferation of a high proportion of lymphocytes from unimmunized mice. These findings were interpreted as providing *"unequivocal evidence that expression of a particular Vβ segment confers preferential T cell reactivity in vitro to Mls-encoded determinants and that TCRs using Vβ6 are selected against in the thymus of mice that express Mls-encoded gene products."* Thus, they felt that, consistent with Burnet's proposal, tolerance is mediated by the deletion of self-reactive clones rather than by alternative mechanisms such as anergy or peripheral suppression.

Very similar findings were reported simultaneously by John Kappler and coworkers.[50]

Although these reports were certainly consistent with Burnet's conjecture that tolerance results from the deletion of immature auto-reactive cells, because specific peptide antigen reactive T cells had not been shown to be deleted, the question remained open. Obviously, the problem was one of detection of very scarce antigen-reactive cells, made impossible by the tremendous diversity of antigen recognition. The development of transgenic mice first in 1980 by Frank Ruddle's group,[51] and then by Ralph Brinster and Richard Palmiter and co-workers ion 1981 and 1982[52,53] provided the necessary tools to analyze the mechanisms responsible for self-tolerance to specific peptide epitopes *in vivo*. Thus, Harald von Boehmer and team took advantage of monoclonal T cells cytolytic for peptides specified by the male minor histocompatability antigen (HY) that they had generated in 1979 using female T cells stimulated by male T cells *in vitro*, and cloned by limiting dilution using IL-2-containing media.[54] They chose one of their clones for study because its TCRβ-chain could be recognized by a monoclonal antibody (MoAb) specific for all three members of the Vβ8 gene family.[55] They then injected fertilized eggs with genomic DNA harboring the productively rearranged TCR α and β genes isolated from the HY-specific cytolytic T cell clone reported a decade later in 1988.[56] The transgenic founder mouse contained four copies of the TCR-α and two copies of the TCR-β transgenes integrated on the same chromosome. Noteworthy, the presence of the transgenes inhibited the expression of the endogenous α and β TCR genes, with the result that the majority of T cells expressed the transgenes.[55] Thus, they essentially created *in vivo* clonal T cells, thereby circumventing the complex TCR repertoire, so that the fate of transgenic T cells expressing only one TCR complex reactive with a single peptide could be studied.

T cells with the phenotype of the cytolytic HY-specific clone were found to be frequent in female, but not in male transgenic offspring, despite that peripheral T cells in animals of both sexes expressed both transgenes. Peripheral T cells in male, but not female mice, had an abnormal CD4/CD8 phenotype, in that over 90% of T cells in the lymph nodes of male transgenic mice lacked the expression of both CD4 and CD8, or expressed very low levels of CD8. Moreover, there were very few CD4+CD8- T cells. This unusual phenotype of peripheral male T cells was a consequence of the deletion of autospecific HY-reactive thymocytes that expressed high densities of CD8 molecules, predominantly cortical CD4+CD8+ immature thymocytes. Therefore, these data supported the interpretation that double-positive cortical thymocytes are precursors of single-positive mature thymocytes, and that the accessory molecules CD4 and CD8 are important for the deletional process. Moreover, these data first established that negative selection of self-peptide-specific T cells occurs because of TCR recognition of self-peptide.

Accordingly, all these data confirmed Burnet's prediction that tolerance to self-autoantigens, at least in the T cell compartment, occurs via the deletion of cells capable of recognizing self-peptides. Moreover, the data from the TCR transgenic mouse experiments were especially convincing that the TCR *and* the accessory molecules, CD4 and CD8, which confer antigenic specificity and sensitivity, were responsible for initiating the deletional process. However, these experiments did not yield any insight into the molecular mechanism(s) operative. In other words, these data revealed "what happens," but they did not provide any clues as to "how it happens."

Negative Selection: Roles of the TCR vs. IL-2 in Triggering Apoptosis

Almost simultaneously, as experiments were reported by investigators focused on genetic approaches in tolerance induction, others were exploring biochemical and immunological approaches to understand T cell maturation and selection in the thymus. Experiments reported in 1985 by David Raulet using flow cytometric analysis revealed that a small thymocyte subpopulation lacks expression of both CD4 and CD8 TCR accessory molecules, and contains the most immature cells (~3% of adult thymocytes). As MoAbs capable of recognizing what is now known as the IL-2Rα chain became available,[57-59] ~1/3 of this "double-negative" thymocyte subpopulation, or only 1% of all thymocytes, were found to express this cytokine receptor chain.[60] In addition, double-negative fetal thymocytes were also positive for IL-2Rα chain expression. Even so, it is noteworthy that when exposed to purified recombinant human IL-2 (rhIL-2), the immature double-negative thymocytes proliferated poorly, thus calling into question whether most of these immature IL-2Ra+ thymocytes expressed a *functional* IL-2R, and also whether IL-2 itself was involved in thymocyte proliferation and differentiation. This was especially cogent, given that Con-A without IL-2 supplementation was ineffective in stimulating thymocyte proliferation, indicating that immature thymocytes could not produce IL-2. Moreover, IL-2Rs were undetectable on the double-positive thymocytes subset, which makes up the majority of immature thymocytes, ~90%, and the stage where negative selection appeared to be taking place.

From 1978 and the earliest experiments with IL-2-dependent CTLL, it was observed that IL-2 deprivation for even a few hours would lead to irreversible cell death, although the mechanism(s) responsible were totally obscure.[61] Accordingly, of interest soon after Raulet's thymocyte experiments, in 1986 Richard Duke and John Cohen reported that IL-2 withdrawal from IL-2-dependent proliferating CTLL and helper T cells results in extensive chromatin cleavage that precedes plasma membrane breakdown by several hours.[62] The DNA fragments observed were not randomly generated but consisted of regular sized oligonucleosomes. Noteworthy was the finding that DNA fragmentation, like cell death, did not occur in the presence of protein synthesis inhibitors, suggesting that IL-2 deprivation leads to the activation of the expression of an endogenous endonuclease specific for linker DNA. All these data indicated that IL-2-deprivation cytolysis occurs via a suicide program with all the classic signs of apoptosis.

A subsequent analysis of murine thymocyte expression of CD3, CD4 and CD8, and reactivity to stimulation via anti-CD3 by James Allison and co-workers in 1987, revealed that 80% of adult thymocytes express both CD4 and CD8 (i.e. double-positive), 3% express neither (double-negative), 12% only express CD4 (CD4 single-positive), and 3% expressed CD8 alone (CD8 single-positive).[63] Noteworthy, there was a distinct difference in CD3 density among the subsets, with the single-positive cells expressing the highest density, while the double-positive cells expressed only a low density of CD3. In this report, only about ½ of the double-positive cells expressed detectable CD3. To assess the functionality of the CD3 signaling molecules expressed by double-positive thymocytes, by comparison with single-positive peripheral T cells isolated from the spleen, single cell intracellular calcium concentrations were measured using flow cytometry. It was obvious that the anti-CD3-triggered increased intracellular Ca^{2+} concentrations of double-positive thymocytes were only about ½ of the mature peripheral splenic T cells. However, PKC, like calcium second messengers, a product of CD3-induced phosphatidylinositol 4,5-bisphosphate hydrolysis, was activated by anti-CD3 stimulation of murine double-positive thymocytes.

As the components of the early steps of T cell activation appeared to be functional in double-positive thymocytes, the expression of the IL-2Rα-chain and the production of IL-2 was assessed next.[63] In contrast to mature peripheral single-positive splenic T cells, the double-positive thymocytes failed to produce IL-2 or to express the IL-2Rα-chain, and to proliferate, even if irradiated macrophages to serve as a source of IL-1 were present. Also, noteworthy was the lack of a proliferative response of the double-positive thymocytes, even if IL-2 was added exogenously, thereby indicating the lack of functional IL-2R expression in response to anti-CD3 stimulation. Accordingly, the CD4CD8 double-positive thymocytes undergo negative selection when triggered via their TCR/CD3 complex by self-peptide/MHC complexes *in vivo*, but the TCR/CD3 complex expressed by these cells appears immature, incapable of promoting transcription and translation of genes such as IL-2 and the IL-2Rα-chain, which are required for a proliferative response by mature peripheral single-positive T cells *in vitro*. ***Thus, a plausible mechanism for the apoptosis underlying negative selection is the lack of IL-2 production and IL-2R expression by TCR/CD3-triggered immature double-positive thymocytes, in that without the IL-2-derived pro-survival and proliferative/differentiative signals, premature TCR/CD3 triggering may well activate apoptosis as a default pathway.***

These data were confirmed and underscored by Ellis Reinherz's group who studied human thymocytes compared with peripheral mature T cells also in 1987.[64] Using the unique observation that CD3-thymocytes could be triggered to proliferate via activation by MoAbs reactive with anti-CD2, they found that anti-CD3 would inhibit this proliferative response. In examining this phenomenon further, they found that CD3+ thymocytes, like their murine counterparts, could not be triggered to proliferate, and that anti-CD3 stimulation did not promote IL-2 production, but did lead to IL-2R expression. Moreover, anti-CD3 activation suppressed IL-2 gene expression stimulated by anti-CD2. Thus, by comparison with mature peripheral T cells, triggering CD3+ thymocytes with anti-CD3 leads to a rapid *suppression* of IL-2 gene expression, thereby preventing the cells from receiving the pro-survival and proliferative effects of IL-2, thus creating a situation imitating cytokine withdrawal apoptosis. Therefore, TCR/CD3 activation of immature thymocytes results in an active suppression of IL-2 gene expression, not simply a passive lack of IL-2 gene activation. This begs the question as to the mechanism responsible, which remained obscure.

This conjecture was supported in 1989 by Eric Jenkinson and John Owens and colleagues, who studied the effects of anti-CD3 on thymocytes in fetal organ culture, which provides an *in vitro* system that can support TCR gene rearrangement and expression, and avoids the problem of low viability encountered in cultures of isolated thymocytes.[65] They found that anti-CD3 added for the last 18 hours of culture resulted in a substantial reduction in cell yield (~43%), and the chromatin condensation and cell shrinkage characteristic of apoptotic cells detectable by electron microscopy, as well as the degradation of DNA to oligonucleosomes characteristic of apoptosis. Similar results were obtained by Owen's group in 1989 using a MoAb reactive with TCR Vβ8, as well as a super-antigen, staphylococcal enterotoxin-B, reactive with TCR Vβ8+ cells. Accordingly, these data are all consistent with the conclusion that triggering of immature CD4CD8 double-positive thymocytes either via MoAbs reactive with CD3, or MoAbs and super-antigens reactive with specific TCR Vβ8+ cells, results in apoptosis rather than activation.[66]

Positive Selection-MHC and Endogenous Peptide

A picture is worth a thousand words, they say, and thus the determination of the structure of human Class I histocompatibility leukocyte antigen (HLA) from crystalized protein by Pamela Bjorkman, working with Donald Wiley and Jack Strominger, rocked the immunological community in 1987.[67] Since the pioneering 1966 experiments of Schlossman[68] and pathbreaking findings of Unanue and Askonas more than 20 years earlier in 1968,[69] it had become established that T cells recognize short peptides (~6–20 residues), digested and presented by antigen presenting cells, somehow complexed to molecules encoded by genes of the major histocompatability complex (MHC).

However, without any knowledge of the structure of these molecules, it was difficult to imagine how the myriad of foreign peptides (estimates of ~ 10^7) could interact with each MHC-encoded molecule, and furthermore, how a single TCR recognized or interacted with the peptide-MHC complex. Accordingly, the shock from visualizing the first HLA molecular structure was finding the peptide-binding groove situated between two alpha helices.[67] Also, finding the groove to be already occupied with what ultimately turned out to be an endogenous peptide that persisted throughout the entire purification and crystallization procedure, suggested that a peptide, either self or nonself, is always bound to the histocompatibility molecules.[70]

Thus, by 1987 it was established that a single TCR recognizes a single peptide-MHC complex, and because of the work of Bjorkman and colleagues, it was finally understood exactly how peptides complexed with the MHC-encoded molecules to form a single peptide/MHC antigen recognition molecule. However, even before the discovery of MHC restriction of T cell antigen recognition, Neils Jerne had proposed that the germ cells carry a set of genes encoding the combining sites of lymphocyte receptors which he hypothesized were directed against a complete set of MHC-encoded antigens of the species to which the animal belongs.[71] Subsequently, it was reported that precursor T cells differentiate recognition structures for self-MHC molecules expressed on the thymic epithelial cells.[72,73] However, exactly how this phenomenon occurred remained obscure.

The two subsets of T cells distinguished by their expression of either CD4 or CD8 molecules were first delineated by Reinherz's group in 1979 and 1980, who studied human peripheral blood mononuclear cells (PBMC),[74,75] and then human IL-2-dependent cytolytic CD8[+] and CD4[+] T cell clones in 1982.[76] Several years after the work with human T cells, a monoclonal antibody that reacts with the murine equivalent of CD4 was developed by Frank Fitch's group, allowing Susan Swain to confirm the correlation between CD4 expression and MHC class II restriction of antigen recognition in the murine system in 1984.[77] Analysis of all of Reinherz's human T cell clones revealed CD8[+] T cells to be MHC Class I restricted, whereas all CD4[+] T cell clones were MHC Class II restricted in their capacity to recognize antigens.[76] Noteworthy from these data was the observation that both MHC Class I restricted and MHC Class II restricted T cell clones were capable of cytolysis as determined by the standard 4-hour ^{51}Cr release assay. However, in addition, CD4[+] MHC Class II restricted T cell clones could also provide T cell "help" for antibody production, and thus could be "helper" T cells (Th). Accordingly, although cytolytic T cells (Tc) were traditionally considered CD8[+] while Th cells considered CD4[+], this discrete separation was not supported by the data derived from T cell clones in 1982.[76] Instead, CD8 expression correlated with MHC Class I antigen recognition, while CD4 expression correlated with MHC Class II antigen recognition.

Thus, it was proposed that mature peripheral thymic-derived cells are somehow "positively selected" from immature thymocytes by MHC-encoded molecules expressed on thymic stromal cells, and upon emerging from the thymus, the TCRs of these cells would bind foreign peptide antigens that are already bound to self-MHC encoded molecules. Accordingly, should this be the case, Harald von Boehmer hypothesized that in the absence of foreign peptides during thymopoiesis, the interaction of the TCR with Class II and Class I thymic self-MHC molecules should direct or select for the differentiation of immature T cells into single-positive CD4[+] and CD8[+] mature T cells, respectively.[78] Thus, von Boehmer's team focused on female TCR transgenic mice that recognized the male-specific HY antigen, because this antigen was absent during thymopoiesis in these animals. Theoretically, female mice should "positively select" CD8⁺ T cells capable of recognizing HY peptide/self MHC, but not self MHC without HY peptide, or HY peptide and a third-party Class I MHC. Their results reported in 1988 were consistent with this hypothesis, i.e. that the interaction of Class I MHC-encoded molecules in the thymus with the αβ heterodimeric TCR determines the CD4/CD8 phenotype of mature T cells in the absence of reactive foreign peptide.[78]

To investigate further the specificity of the "positive selection" exerted by MHC-encoded molecules, the von Boehmer team performed thymus repopulation experiments reported in 1988[79]: lethally irradiated females of recombinant strains that differed at D and K through to the S sub-regions of the MHC, were transplanted with bone marrow cells from H-2^b TCR αβ HY-specific transgenic female mice. Five weeks after transplantation, the repopulating capacity of the donor stem cells, as estimated from the cellularity of the thymuses of the recipients, correlated with the degree of compatibility within the MHC: the highest numbers of thymocytes ($\sim 5 \times 10^7$) were recovered from syngeneic and semi-allogeneic recipients, the lowest ($\sim 8 \times 10^6$) from allogeneic recipients differing across the whole MHC. These investigators went on to hypothesize "*that the specific low affinity interaction of the TCR with thymic stromal MHC-encoded molecules is sufficient to select immature T cells but insufficient to activate mature T cells. The specific low affinity interaction in the thymus may be complemented by accessory molecules* (CD4/CD8 co-receptors) *present on either immature thymocytes or selecting thymic stromal cells, or both. Such a complementation could then lead to the positive selection of T cells with low affinity for self-MHC.*"

Entirely consistent with these findings and hypothesis, von Boehmer's group followed up their *in vivo* findings with *in vitro* experiments using double-positive thymocytes from female H-2^b TCR αβ HY-specific transgenic mice. When exposed to thymic or splenic adherent cells from male H-2^b mice during 24–48 hours of suspension culture, deletion of double-positive female thymocytes occurred only in the presence of cells bearing HY antigen with the appropriate (H-2^b) MHC-encoded molecules. These findings indicated that the deletion of double-positive thymocytes is not a unique property of the thymic microenvironment, but is the property of a certain developmental stage of T cells, which makes it sensitive to deletion. Thus, female double-positive thymocytes will be deleted when exposed to the HY-antigen presented by the proper MHC-encoded molecules *in vitro*, just as the male double-positive thymocytes are deleted *in vivo*, when exposed to their own self-antigen. Also noteworthy is the fact that female single-positive CD8$^+$ mature peripheral T cells do not undergo apoptosis when confronted with HY$^+$ APCs. Rather, they undergo activation and clonal expansion, underscoring the interpretation that immature double-positive thymocytes are negatively selected because of their immaturity.

It is also noteworthy that the hypothesis to explain these findings of positive and negative selection, i.e. that there must be a difference in the *affinity* of self-antigen stimulation of the TCR-co-accessory molecular complex to account for such disparate fates of life vs. death, remained untested at the time in the early 1990s. A further, unexplored aspect of positive selection is the question of whether, like negative selection, a self-peptide occupies the groove of the MHC-encoded molecules in the thymus, such that all the positively selected T cells that exit the thymus and populate the periphery have the capacity of reacting to self, should the self-peptide concentration become high enough to surpass a putative threshold, leading to T cell activation, proliferative clonal expansion and differentiation to become effector cells capable of autoimmune reactivity. Alternatively, perhaps there is a peripheral tolerance mechanism that functions to prevent auto-recognition and activation. These considerations would necessarily be the subjects of future investigations.

In the decade after the discovery of the molecular nature of the TCR complex and the realization that T cell effector molecules are antigen nonspecific leukocytotrophic hormones, it was possible to begin to identify, isolate and characterize the molecules responsible for adaptive immunity for the first time. Thus, the biochemical analysis of antigen-specific TCR signaling revealed that lymphocytes are excitable cells, not too different from neuromuscular cells, that react to their molecular environment by signaling through their lipid membranes, leading to ion fluxes and activation of phosphorylating enzyme cascades that regulate the genetic expression of the cells. Among the first and most important of the molecules encoded by the genes activated by the TCR were the molecules involved in cytolysis and helper functions. The biochemical understanding of apoptosis provided a molecular process by which negative selection of immature lymphocytes reactive with self-molecules provided a firm molecular underpinning of Burnet's prediction that self-reactive clones would be eliminated during development. T cell clones and cloned TCR genes permitted the generation of transgenic animals that were instrumental in demonstrating that the phenomena of negative and positive selection occur.

References

1. Nowell PC. (1960). Phytohemagglutinin: An initiator of mitosis in cultures of normal human leukocytes. *Cancer Res* **20**:462–468.
2. Deutsch C, Holian A, Holian S, *et al.* (1979). Transmembrane electrical and pH gradients across human erythrocytes and human peripheral lymphocytes. *J Cell Physiol* **99**:79–93.
3. Tsien R, Pouzzan T and Rink T. (1982). T-cell mitogens cause early changes in cytoplasmic free Ca2+ and membrane potential in lymphocytes. *Nature* **295**:68–71.
4. Nishizuka Y. (1980). Three multifunctional protein kinase systems in transmembrane control. *Mol Biol Biochem Biophys* **32**:113–135.
5. Nishizuka Y. (1984). Turnover of inositol phospholipids and signal transduction. *Science* **225**:1365–1370.
6. Weiss M, Daley J, Hodgdon J and Reinherz EL. (1984). Calcium dependency of antigen-specific (T3-Ti) and alternative pathways of human T cell activation. *Proc Natl Acad Sci USA* **81**:6836–6840.
7. Gillis S and Watson J. (1980). Biochemical and biological characterization of lymphocyte regulatory molecules. *J Exp Med* **152**:1709–1719.
8. Robb RJ and Smith KA. (1981). Heterogeneity of human T-cell growth factor(s) due to variable glycosylation. *Mol Immunol* **18**:1087–1094.

9. Weiss A, Wiskocil R and Stobo J. (1984). The role of T3 surface molecules in the activation of human cells: A two-stimulus requirement for iL-2 production reflects events occurring at a pretranslational level. *J Immunol* **133**:123–128.

10. Weiss A, Imboden J, Shoback D and Stobo J. (1984). Role of T3 surface molecules in human T cell activation: T3-dependent activation results in an increase in cytoplasmic free calcium. *Proc Natl Acad Sci USA* **81**:4169–4173.

11. Brunner KT, Mauel J, Cerottini J-C and Chapius B. (1968). Quantitative assay of the lytic action of lymphoid cells on 51-Cr labelled allogeneic target cells *in vitro*. Inhibition by isoantibody and drugs. *Immunology* **14**:181–190.

12. Dourmashkin R, Deteix P, Simone C and Henkart P. (1980). Electron microscopic demonstration of lesions in target cell membranes associated with antibody-dependent cellular cytotoxicity. *Clin Exp Immunol* **42**:554–560.

13. Podack E and Dennert G. (1983). Assembly of two types of tubules with putative cytolytic function by cloned natural killer cells. *Nature* **302**:442–445.

14. Dennert G and Podack E. (1983). Cytolysis by H-2-specific T killer cells: Assembly of tubular complexes on target membranes. *J Exp Med* **157**:1483–1495.

15. Gillis S and Smith KA. (1977). Long term culture of tumour-specific cytotoxic T cells. *Nature* **268**:154–156.

16. Baker PE, Gillis S and Smith KA. (1979). Monoclonal cytolytic T-cell lines. *J Exp Med* **149**:273–278.

17. Podack ER and Koningsberg PJ. (1984). Cytolytic T cell granules. Isolation, structural, biochemical, and functional characterization. *J Exp Med* **160**:695–710.

18. Henkart P, Millard P, Reynolds C and Henkart M. (1984). Cytolytic activity of purified cytoplasmic granules from cytotoxic rat large granular lymphocyte tumors. *J Exp Med* **160**:75–93.

19. Podack ER, Young JD and Cohn ZA. (1985). Isolation and biochemical and functional characterization of peforin 1 from cytolytic T cell granules. *Proc Natl Acad Sci USA* **82**:8629–8633.

20. Masson D and Tschopp J. (1985). Isolation of a lytic, pore-forming protein (perforin) from cytolytic T lymphocytes. *J Biol Chem* **260**:9069–9072.

21. Young J, Cohn Z and Podack E. (1986). The ninth component of complement and the pore-forming protein (perforin 1) from cytolytic T cells: Structural, immunological, and functional similarities. *Science* **233**:184–190.

22. Lowrey D, Aebischer T, Olsen K, et al. (1989). Cloning, analysis, and expression of murine perforin 1 cDNA, a component of cytolytic granules with homology to complement component C9. Proc Natl Acad Sci USA 86:247–251.

23. Chang T and Eisen H. (1980). Effects of N-Tosyl-L-Lysysl-chloro-methylketone on the activity of cyttoxic T lymphocytes. J Immunol 124:1028–1033.

24. Pasternack M and Eisen H. (1985). A novel serine esterase expressed by cytotoxic T lymphocytes. Nature 314:743–745.

25. Lobe C, Havele C and Bleackley R. (1986). Cloning of two genes that are specifically expressed in activated T lymphocytes. Proc Natl Acad Sci USA 83:1448–1452.

26. Gershenfeld H and Weissman I. (1986). Cloning of a cDNA for a T cell-specific serine protease from a cytotoxic T lymphocyte. Science 232:854–858.

27. Lobe C, Finlay L, Paranchych W, et al. (1986). Novel serine proteases encoded by two cytotoxic T lymphocyte-specific genes. Science 232:858–861.

28. Masson D and Tschopp J. (1987). A family of serine esterases in lytic granules of cytolytic T lymphocytes. Cell 49:679–685.

29. Kerr J, Wyllie A and Currie A. (1972). Apoptosis: A basic biological phenomenon with wide-ranging implications in tissue kinetics. Br J Cancer 26:239–257.

30. Russell J, Masakowski V and Dobos C. (1980). Mechanisms of immune lysis: I. Physiological distinction between target cell death mediated by cytotoxic T lymphocytes and antibody plus complement. J Immunol 124:1100–1105.

31. Russell J and Dobos C. (1980). Mechanisms of immune lysis: II. CTL-induced nuclear disintegartion of the target begins within minutes of cell contact. J Immunol 125:1256–1261.

32. Duke R, Chervenak R and Cohen J. (1983). Endogenous endonuclease-induced DNA fragmentation: An early event in cell-mediated cytolysis. Proc Natl Acad Sci USA 80:6361–6365.

33. Hayes M, Berrebi G and Henkart P. (1989). Induction of target cell DNA release by the cytotoxic T lymphocyte granule protease Granzyme A. J Exp Med 170:933–946.

34. Shi L, Kraut R, Aebersold R and Greenberg A. (1992). A Natural Killer cell granule protein that induces DNA fragmentation and apoptosis. J Exp Med 175:553–566.

35. Owen R. (1945). Immunogenetic consequences of vascular anastomoses between bovine twins. *Science* **102**:400–401.

36. Billingham RE, Brent L and Medawar PB. (1953). Actively acquired tolerance of foreign cells. *Nature* **172**:603–606.

37. Burnet F and Fenner F. (1949). *Production of Antibodies.* Melbourne: MacMillan.

38. Burnet FM. (1959). *The Clonal Selection Theory of Acquired Immunity.* Cambridge: Cambridge University Press.

39. Miller J. (1962). Effect of neonatal thymectomy on the immunological responsiveness of the mouse. *Proc Roy Soc Lond-B* **156**:415–428.

40. Cooper M, Peterson R and Good R. (1965). Delineation of the thymic and bursal lymphoid systems in the chicken. *Nature* **205**:143–146.

41. Cooper M, Peterson R, South M and Good R. (1966). The functions of the thymus system and the bursa system in the chicken. *J Exp Med* **123**:75–102.

42. Raff M, Sternberg M and Taylor RB. (1970). Immunoglobulin determinants on the surface of mouse lymphoid cells. *Nature* **225**:553–555.

43. Pernis B, Forni L and Amante L. (1970). Immunoglobulin spots on the surface of rabbit lymphocytes. *J Exp Med* **132**:1001–1018.

44. Meuer SC, Fitzgerald KA, Hussey RE, *et al.* (1983). Clonotypic structures involved in antigen-specific human T cell function. Relationship to the T3 molecular complex. *J Exp Med* **157**:705–719.

45. Meuer S, Acuto O, Hussey R, *et al.* (1983). Evidence for the T3-associated 90K heterodimer as the T cell antigen receptor. *Nature* **303**:808–810.

46. Meuer S, Cooper D, Hodgdon J, *et al.* (1983). Identification of the receptor for antigen and major histocompatability complex on human inducer T lymphocytes. *Science* **222**:1239–1242.

47. Kappler J, Wade T, White J, *et al.* (1987). A T cell receptor V-beta segment that imparts reactivity to a class II major histocompatibility complex product. *Cell* **49**:263–271.

48. Kappler J, Roehm N and Marrack P. (1987). T cell tolerance by clonal elimination in the thymus. *Cell* **49**:273–280.

49. MacDonald H, Schneider R, Lees R, *et al.* (1988). T-cell receptor V-beta use predicts reactivity and tolerance to Mls-encoded antigens. *Nature* **332**.

50. Kappler J, Staerz U, White J and Marrack P. (1988). Self-tolerance eliminates T cells specific for Mls-modified products of the major histocompatibility complex. *Nature* **332**:35–40.

51. Gordon J, Scangos G, Plotkin D and Ruddle F. (1980). Genetic transformation of mouse embryos by microinjection of purified DNA. *Proc Natl Acad Sci USA* **77**:7380–7384.

52. Brinster R, Chen H, Trumbauer M, *et al.* (1981). Somatic expression of herpes thymidine kinase in mice following injection of a fusion gene into eggs. *Cell* **27**:223–231.

53. Brinster R, Chen H, Warren R, *et al.* (1982). Regulation of metallothionein-thymidine kinase fusion plasmids injected into mouse eggs. *Nature* **296**:39–42.

54. von Boehmer H, Hengartner H, Nabholz M, *et al.* (1979). Fine specificity of a continuously growing killer cell clone specific for H-Y antigen. *Eur J Immunol* **9**:592–597.

55. Uematsu Y, Ryser S, Dembic Z, *et al.* (1988). In transgenic mice the introduced functional T cell receptor beta gene prevents expression of endogenous beta genes. *Cell* **52**:831–841.

56. Kisielow P, Bluthmann H, Staerz U, *et al.* (1988). Tolerance in T-cell-receptor transgenic mice involves deletion of nonmature CD4⁺8⁺ thymocytes. *Nature* **333**:742–746.

57. Leonard WJ, Depper JM, Uchiyama T, *et al.* (1982). A monoclonal antibody that appears to recognize the receptor for human T-cell growth factor; partial characterization of the receptor. *Nature* **300**:267–269.

58. Malek T, Robb R and Shevach E. (1983). Identification and initial characterization of a rat monoclonal antibody reactive with the murine interleukin-2 receptor ligand complex. *Proc Natl Acad Sci USA* **80**:5694–5698.

59. Ortega G, Robb R, Shevach E and Malek T. (1984). The murine IL-2 receptor. I. Monoclonal antibodies that define distinct functional epitopes on activated T cells and react with activated B cells. *J Immunol* **133**:1970–1975.

60. Raulet D. (1985). Expression and function of interleukin-2 receptor on immature thymocytes. *Nature* **314**:101–103.

61. Gillis S, Ferm MM, Ou W and Smith KA. (1978). T cell growth factor: Parameters of production and a quantitative microassay for activity. *J Immunol* **120**:2027–2032.

62. Duke R and Cohen J (1986). IL-2 addiction: Withdrawal of growth factor activates a suicide program in dependent T cells. *Lymphokine Res* **5**:289–299.

63. Havran W, Poenie M, Kimura J, *et al.* (1987) Expression and function of the CD3-antigen receptor on murine CD4+CD8+ thymocytes. *Nature* **300**.

64. Ramarli D, Fox D and Reinherz E. (1987). Selective inhibition of interleukin-2 gene function following thymocyte antigen/major histocompatibility complex receptor crosslinking: Possible thymic selection mechanism. *Proc Natl Acad Sci USA* **84**:8598–8602.
65. Smith C, Williams G, Kingston R, et al. (1989). Antibodies to CD3/T-cell receptor complex induce death by apoptosis in immature T cells in thymic cultures. *Nature* **337**:181–184.
66. Jenkinson E, Kingston R, Smith C, et al. (1989). Antigen-induced apoptosis in developing T cells: A mechanism for negative selection of the T cell receptor repertoire. *Eur J Immunol* **19**:2175–2177.
67. Bjorkman PJ, Saper MA, Samaoui B, et al. (1987). Structure of the human class I histocompatability antigen, HLA-A2. *Nature* **329**:506–511.
68. Schlossman S, Ben-Efraim S, Yaron A and Sober H. (1966). Immunochemical studies on the antigenic determinants required to elicit delayed and immediate hypersensitivity reactions. *J Exp Med* **123**: 1083–1095.
69. Unanue E and Askonas BA. (1968). Persistence of immunogenicity of antigen after uptake by macrophages. *J Exp Med* **127**.
70. Bjorkman P, Saper M, Samaraoui B, et al. (1987). The foreign antigen binding site and T cell recognition regions of class I histocompatability antigens. *Nature* **329**:512–518.
71. Jerne NK. (1971). The somatic generation of immune recognition. *Eur J Immunol* **1**:1–9.
72. Zinkernagel R, Callahan G, Althage A, et al. (1978). On the thymus in the differentiation of "H-2 self recognition" by T cells: Evidence for dual recognition? *J Exp Med* **147**:882–896.
73. von Boehmer H, Haas W and Jerne N. (1978). Major histocompatibility comples-linked immune responsiveness is acquired by lymphocytes of low responder mice differentiating in thymus of high responder mice. *Proc Natl Acad Sci USA* **75**:2439–2442.
74. Reinherz E, Kung P, Goldstein G and Schlossman S. (1979). Further characterization of the human inducer T cell subset defined by monoclonal antibody. *J Immunol* **123**:2894–2896.
75. Reinherz E, Kung P, Goldstein G and Schlossman S. (1980). A monoclonal antibody reactive with the human cytotoxic/suppressor T cell subset previously defined by a heteroantiserum termed TH2. *J Immunol* **124**:1301–1307.
76. Meuer S, Schlossman S and Reinherz E. (1982). Clonal analysis of human cytolytic T lymphocytes: T4+ and T8+ effector T cells recognize

products of different major histocompatibility regions. *Proc Natl Acad Sci USA* **79**:4395–4399.

77. Swain S, Dialynas D, Fitch F and English M. (1984). Monoclonal antibody to L3T4 blocks the function of T cells specific for class 2 major histocompatibility complex antigens. *J Immunol* **132**:1118–1123.

78. Teh H, Kisielow P, Scott B, *et al.* (1988). Thymic major histocompatibility complex antigens and the alpha beta T-cell receptor determine the CD4/CD8 phenotype of T cells. *Nature* **335**:229–233.

79. Kisielow P, Teh H, Bluthmann H and H vB. (1988). Positive selection of antigen-specific T cells in thymus by restricting MHC molecules. *Nature* **335**:730–733.

5 Molecular Mechanisms of T Cell "Help"

Interleukins

One of the purposes of the creation of the interleukin nomenclature, whereby the molecules were simply numbered, was the anticipation of additional new and novel interleukins yet to be discovered. In this regard, murine Th clones had already been generated using CATSUP by Max Schreier and co-workers in 1980.[1,2] Thus, operating with the hypothesis that there must be a Th cell-specific growth factor or interleukin similar but different from the CTL-specific IL-2, Andrew Hapel working in James Ihle's group, reported in 1980 that a new and novel cytokine promoted the proliferation and differentiation of immature hematopoietic precursor cells of athymic (*nu/nu*) to become Lyt-1+Lyt2- Th cells.[3] However, these investigators appeared to be unaware that the Lyt-1 alloantigen, which had been thought to mark Th cells, had been found also in 1980 by Leonard Herzenberg's group on all T cells,[4] so that Lyt1 did not specify the Th subset as did the CD4 molecule expressed by human T cells.[4,5] In any event, since IL-2 appeared to preferentially lead to the growth of CTL at the time, it seemed reasonable that there might also by a Th-specific growth and differentiation factor in CATSUP. Ihle's group had also reported in 1981 that conditioned media from mitogen- or alloantigen-stimulated lymphocytes promoted the expression of 20a-hydroxysteroid dehydrogenase, which had been reported to be associated with mature but not immature T cells.[6,7] Because this activity in CATSUP appeared to target immature hematopoietic cells, and because the initial biochemical characteristics of the activity appeared to be different from those reported for both IL-1 and IL-2, Ihle's group proposed that the activity be termed IL-3. Of course, all this occurred before any cytokine activity had been purified to homogeneity and attributed to a single molecule, so this proposed nomenclature was problematic and premature.

Unbeknownst to Hapel and Ihle, John Schrader had also reported in 1981 that CATSUP promoted the outgrowth of immunoglobulin-negative, Thy-1-negative and Lyt1/Lyt2-negative non-adherent cells from murine splenocytes, which he termed "persisting cells" (P-cells).[8] By comparison with the lack of these T cell markers, MHC-encoded Class I and II molecules as well as Fc receptors were readily detected on these cells. In other experiments, metachromatic granules were found in these cells, and they were found to contain histamine, suggesting that the P cells were from the mast cell lineage.[9] Schrader went on to show in 1982 that the activity that he found in CATSUP was similar to the colony stimulating activity (CSA) described by Donald Metcalf and colleagues that promoted the growth of mixed hematopoietic colonies of erythroid and myeloid cells, but was distinct from T cell growth factor (TCGF) and T cell-derived granulocyte-macrophage colony-stimulating factor (GM-CSF).[10]

Soon thereafter, in 1984 Hapel and co-workers reported the cloning of a cDNA encoding murine IL-3, which they identified by the growth promoting effects of oocyte-translated mRNA on an IL-3-dependent cell line 32D clone-23 created by Ihle's group.[11] The nucleotide sequence predicted an amino acid sequence with a molecular size of 15,102 Da, so that it was similar but not identical to IL-2.[12,13] Hapel's group then collaborated with Metcalf's group in 1985 to show that the molecularly cloned IL-3 induced 20α-hydroxysteroid dehydrogenase activity in splenic lymphocytes from athymic (nu/nu) mice, in addition to proliferative activity for 32D clone-23 and FDC-P1 cell lines, and CSA for granulocyte-macrophage, eosinophil, megakaryocyte, natural killer-like, erythroid and multipotential colony-forming cells from murine fetal liver and adult bone marrow.[14] Thus, IL-3 was shown to promote multipotential hematopoietic stem cell proliferation, and not to be a Th-specific growth factor.

As detailed in Chapters 1 and 2, at least three cell types were found to be required for the generation of antibody forming cells

(AFCs) *in vitro;* B cells, T cells and macrophages. Avrion Mitchison had shown in 1971 that there appeared to be a "linked or cognate recognition" between B cells and helper T cells important for the mechanism of T cell help leading to the generation of AFCs.[15] Also, the contribution of both macrophages and T cells could largely be replaced by supernatants from these cultured cells,[16,17] so that there seemed to be both cell-associated and soluble components to the "help" that B cells received from T cells and macrophages. Subsequently, during the 1970s, many purported to show either macrophage- or T cell-derived soluble helper activities that promoted the generation of AFCs, either by promoting B cell proliferation or Ig secretion or both. However, because of the complexities of target cell populations used in the bioassays, as well as the difficulties of protein analysis and purification, and the intricacies of monitoring both proliferation and Ig secretion, the field did not progress for more than a decade.

With the advent of the generation of both cytolytic and helper T cell clones in 1979 and 1980,[1,18] the stage was set for reductionist science to approach the question of the molecular regulation of AFC generation and the contributions of both macrophages and T cells. In particular, Max Schreier and co-workers generated multiple Th clones specific for sheep red blood cells (SRC) or horse red blood cells (HRC) as antigens that were amenable to the analysis of their effects on AFCs using the Jerne plaque assay[19] and the the Mishell-Dutton system.[20] Early on, they established that antigen-specific Th cell clones, propagated in culture in serum-free medium for up to 15 months, would enable *nu/nu* mice to respond to T-dependent antigens *in vivo* by producing specific antibodies and the formation of as much as five-times the number of AFCs as expected in a primary response of normal mice.[1]

Schreier then went on to examine the nature of T cell help. In a detailed analysis of T cell help using Th clones, and as targets either LPS-activated B cell blasts or isolated small resting B cells, they found that Th clones released an antigen/APC-activated MHC Class II-restricted "soluble helper factor" that promoted LPS-induced B cell blast proliferation and Ig secretion.[21,22] This soluble "T cell helper factor" was effective regardless of the MHC or antigen specificity of the B cell blasts. By comparison, small resting B cells required the physical presence of Th clones, as well as their antigen/MHC-restricted antigen-nonspecific secreted soluble Th factor to undergo proliferative expansion and Ig secretion. It appeared that small resting B cells needed two signals, one of which is derived from the Th-B cell contact from Th antigen "linked recognition" to become responsive to the soluble Th factor, which then promoted proliferation.

Several aspects of these results warrant analysis. First, the generation of B cell blasts for use as target cells introduced an unknown, in that at the time the nature of the LPS-induced blastogenesis and proliferation remained obscure. It was not at all clear why LPS was a B cell mitogen in the mouse but not in the human,[23] and whether LPS mimicked antigen-activation or not. Secondly, these experiments were performed before the molecular nature of the TCR was realized, and before the nature of peptide antigen binding to MHC-encoded molecules on APCs was known. Thus, these investigators conjectured that the "linked or cognate" antigen recognition occurred via antigen bound to surface Ig on the B cell (B cell antigen receptor, BCR) and antigen bound to the TCR on the surface of the T cell, as proposed originally by Mitchison in 1971.[15] However, in addition, they suggested that a second signal was supplied to the B cell by the T cell, via the elusive 2nd TCR interacting with B cell Class II MHC-encoded molecules. Despite these complexities and unknowns, the data generated using Th clones and B cell blasts vs. small resting B cells were irrefutable and had to be explained.

The cellular source, as well as the molecular nature of Schreier's antigen-nonspecific B cell replication and maturation factor (BRMF) was obscure. Thus, the investigators stated that the cellular source of the factor "*may be either the antigen-specific helper T cell or the macrophages that interact with the helper T cell.*" Also, "*We imply that one factor* (molecule) *induces both maturation* (i.e. Ig production) *and* (DNA) *replication, although it is equally possible that separate factors* (molecules) *govern these two reactions of a B cell.*" This same interpretation was applied in a separate 1980 report by Schreier that explored the various soluble factors produced by Th clones.[24] When Th clones were stimulated by specific antigen and histocompatible APCs, several apparently distinct activities appeared in culture supernatants that promoted colony formation of various hematopoietic cells, including macrophages, granulocytes, erythroid cells, as well as TCGF and BCGF activities. However, even though Th clones were used rather than heterogeneous T cell populations, because heterogeneous APCs + antigens were required to elicit the activities, the cellular source of each of these activities remained unknown, i.e. whether T cell or macrophage derived, and whether there were many or only one cell and molecule responsible.

Taking a page from the TCGF/IL-2 experience, the use of cloned Th cells at least solved the problem of the identity of the T cells used to produce the conditioned media containing the active molecules. However, long-term normal B cell lines and clones had yet to be developed, so that the target B cells used for the bioassays were still heterogeneous. Therefore, the next best approach was to use B cell blasts obtained using activation with B cell mitogens, or alternatively, B lymphoma cells, which could be cloned. In 1981, Ellen Pure, working in Ellen Vitetta's group, in collaboration with Gunther Dennert, Susan Swain, Richard Dutton and Kyoshi Takatsu, studied the effects of T cell supernatants obtained from a normal alloantigen-specific T cell line, as well as Con-A-activated T cell lymphoma and hybridoma cells, on the proliferation and polyclonal IgM production by anti-IgM/D-activated neonatal and adult splenocytes as well as BCL_1 lymphoma cells.[25] They found that Sepharose-bound anti-Ig induced the proliferation of adult but not neonatal B cells, and that IgM production required T cell supernatants, which induced the production of IgM by both normal (neonatal and adult) and neoplastic B cells. These data seemed to indicate that BCR stimulation led to proliferation, but that differentiation to Ig production depended upon factors in the T cell supernatants.

In a separate 1981 report, Susan Swain and Richard Dutton examined T cell replacing factor (TRF) activity derived from the same alloantigen-stimulated long-term T cell line generated by Gunther Dennert.[26] Using the classic TRF assay of Schimpl and Wecker, comprising of SRBCs cultured with T- and macrophage-depleted splenocytes[17] as a source of target B cells, they found that supernatants from this T cell line had TRF activity but not IL-1 or IL-2 activity. Of note, this TRF supernatant synergized with IL-2 in the generation of AFCs, which was especially evident when the two activities were titrated. They speculated that this activity could be the "late-acting TRF," originally described by Schimpl and Wecker, which was postulated to replace the requirement for T cells by promoting the differentiation of antigen-stimulated B cells, facilitating the production of IgM. However, these investigators rightly discussed the problems associated with the interpretations of their experiments, which used heterogeneous cell populations and T cell lines instead of cloned cells. For example, any soluble activity might amplify residual T cells in the purified B cell population instead of working directly on the B cells themselves. In addition, in the early 1980s, no biochemical characterizations of the TRF activity were reported.

Soon thereafter, Peter Krammer and Ellen Vitetta reported evidence for "B cell differentiation factor(s)" (BCDFs), which appeared to promote B cells to switch isotypes from IgM to IgG (from ~1% to ~20% of AFCs), and especially to IgG_1 (from ~40% to ~90%).[27] As targets, they used LPS splenic B cell blasts purified by negative selection with monoclonal anti-Thy1 + complement (C'), plus supernatants from two long-term IL-2-dependent alloreactive T cell lines stimulated with Con-A. B cells cultured for six days with LPS and T cell supernatant wielded IgG AFCs, whereas no IgG AFCs were produced by LPS alone, only IgM AFCs. These T cell supernatants promoted the appearance of IgG from fluorescent activated cell sorter (FACS)-selected IgG-negative B cells, and furthermore, a switch from IgG_{2a} and IgG_{2b}/IgG_3 to predominantly IgG_1 (~90%) occurred. They speculated that the LPS-dependence of Ig production of any isotype at all suggested the necessity for a specific signal that could have been a proliferative signal or one that induced the expression of receptors for the BCDF(s). By means of the traditional IL-2 and TRF assays, it was determined that the supernatants from the two T cell lines were negative, so that it was concluded that they had identified a new activity, even though they provided no data regarding molecular characteristics.

Simultaneously, Maureen Howard working in William Paul's group, in collaboration with John Farrar and Kiyoshi Takatsu, reported in 1982 the identification of a T cell-derived B cell growth factor (BCGF) distinct from IL-2,[28] based on a system that David Parker had reported in 1980.[29] By comparison with the assays of others, this group used as targets negatively-selected (various antibodies reactive with T cells + C') splenic B cells activated for 72 hours with affinity-purified goat anti-mouse IgM. For a source of T cell activities, supernatants were obtained from a mouse thymoma (EL4) and a T cell hybridoma activated with phorbol myristic acetate (PMA) for 48 hours. PMA was removed from the supernatants by absorption with activated charcoal. As in the IL-2 bioassay, the relative concentrations of BCGF activities were compared by the reciprocal of the dilution that yielded 50% of maximal activity. When 50 µg/mL of anti-IgM was used with 5×10^5 cells/microwell, an easily detectable proliferative response could be quantified with ^{3}H-TdR incorporation without the addition of a T cell supernatant. However, at 10-fold lower anti-IgM concentrations and cell densities, T cell supernatants were required to promote detectable ^{3}H-TdR incorporation. To exclude the possibility that IL-2 was responsible for the BCGF activity, the supernatants were absorbed with cloned IL-2-dependent T cells. Moreover, molecular gel filtration of the supernatants yielded distinct peaks of IL-2 and BCGF activities. Both partially purified IL-2 and BCGF failed to replace the requirement for T cells in the generation of AFCs from purified B cells + SRBCs (TRF activity). However, the inclusion of all three activities (IL-2, BCGF and TRF) did yield AFCs. Thus, these investigators concluded that these three activities functioned independently to promote B cell proliferation and differentiation to AFCs. Like our 1980 model of T cell activation and proliferation,[30,31] these investigators proposed *"that anti-IgM delivers a non-proliferative signal to resting B cells, possibly causing the expression of receptors for BCGF; and that BCGF delivers a proliferative signal to these anti-Ig-activated growth factor-sensitive B cells."*

In collaboration with Steven Mizel and Lawrence Lachman, Maureen Howard and William Paul went on to show in 1983 that in addition to triggering the BCRs, optimal B cell proliferation required both a T cell-derived BCGF and a late-acting signal derived from purified IL-1.[32] From their experiments, it was shown that this combination would only result in B cell proliferation and not Ig secretion, and furthermore that the target B cells had to be cultured at low cell densities (5×10^4 cells/well or 2.5×10^5 cells/mL) for the BCGF and IL-1 effects to become detectable. It did not appear that the IL-1 acted by stimulating residual T cells to produce another BCGF similar to the effect of IL-1 on T cells to produce IL-2,[33,34] but the mechanism of the IL-1 B cell proliferative effect remained unexplored.

In 1983, Susan Swain and Richard Dutton collaborated with Maureen Howard, as well as John Kappler, Philippa Marrack and James Watson, to try to discern whether there were several or only one T cell-derived BCGF.[35] They found that supernatants derived from the EL4 thymoma synergized with anti-Ig in promoting the proliferation of normal splenic B cells, but failed to have activity when the BCL$_1$ lymphoma cells were the target. This activity they termed BCGF-I. By comparison, supernatants from the Dennert alloreactive T cell line had reciprocal activities, promoting the proliferation of BCL$_1$ cells, but not anti-Ig-stimulated normal splenic B cells (BCGF-II). They discussed the conundrum of wondering whether there were different states of B cell differentiation responsive to different growth factors, or whether there were different subsets of B cells involved. Again, a molecular characterization of the activities was lacking. However, they went on to show that homogeneous, MoAb-purified IL-2 acted on an antigen-specific (ovalbumin) T cell line to produce BCGF-I, thereby indicating that the various cytokine activities found in antigen-activated T cell supernatants could very well be interdependent.[36]

In 1985 Paschalis Sideras, working in Eva Severinson's group on the IgG$_1$-inducing factor, constructed a quantitative bioassay patterned after the TCGF bioassay using normal LPS-stimulated splenocytes as target cells and isotype-specific AFCs as the indicators.[37] This assay yielded parallel dose-response curves identical to those described for the TCGF assay, and the relative concentrations obtained from different IL-2-dependent cloned alloreactive T cells or hybridomas stimulated with Con-A could be ascertained by the 50%

AFC responses. Using this assay, they found that the IgG_1 inducing activity, and the IgG_3/IgG_{2b} reducing activities, co-migrated both quantitatively and qualitatively, thereby suggesting that they were attributable to the same lymphokine activity. Furthermore, preparations of BCGF-I, purified by Ohara and Paul via MoAb affinity[38] scored positive in their IgG_1 inducing bioassay, as well as the IgG_1 inducing assay of Vitetta. Accordingly, these data suggested that a single molecule might be responsible for both B cell proliferative (BCGF) and differentiative (BCDF) activities. Moreover, the biochemical properties of this activity differed from those reported for IL-1, IL-2, IL-3, CSA, IFNg, BCGF-II, and TRF.[39]

To proceed beyond these experimental approaches, Severinson collaborated with Tasuku Honjo's group in 1986 to identify a cDNA encoding a protein with IgG_1 inducing activity.[40] The cDNA predicted a protein of 140 amino acid residues and a deduced $M_r = 15,836$, with a signal peptide of 19 residues. Thus, the predicted mature polypeptide had a $M_r = 14,137$ and a sequence distinct from known cytokines, including IL-1, IL-2, IL-3, GM-CSF, and $IFN_{\alpha\beta\gamma}$. Biological assays indicated that IgG_1-inducing activity, $IgG_{2/3}$-reducing activity, B cell Ia-inducing activity and BCGF-I activity were all attributable to the same protein. Accordingly, these investigators proposed that this activity be termed IL-4. An identical cDNA was isolated by Frank Lee and co-workers in Ken-Ichi Arai's group, who also showed that this new lymphokine had TCGF and mast cell growth factor activities, as well as IgE inducing activity.[41]

Others working contemporaneously focused on TRF activity and BCGF-II activity, trying to understand exactly how many lymphokine molecules were involved in promoting B cell proliferation and differentiation. Like the evolution of IL-3, which eventually was found to have growth factor activity for multipotential hematopoietic cells, Colin Sanderson, Gerry Klaus and co-workers found in 1986 that an eosinophil differentiating factor (EDF) also promoted the growth and differentiation of BCL_1 lymphoma cells, thereby suggesting that a single might target both myeloid and lymphoid cells.[42] Their evidence derived from a significant correlation between the EDF and BCGF-II assays when supernatants from 39 separate T cell clones were tested, as well as coincidence in gel filtration and HPLC elution profiles. Subsequently, Kiyoshi Takatsu and Eva Severinson collaborated with Tasuku Honjo's group, and identified a cDNA clone that coded for 133 amino acid residues containing a 21 residue leader sequence and a mature protein of $M_r = 12,300$.[43] The entire amino acid sequence was unique, but contained short sequences homologous to those of IL-3, GM-CSF and IFNγ, thereby suggesting that it belonged to a cytokine family. Because this new and novel protein demonstrated both TRF and BCGF-II activities, it was proposed to be termed IL-5.

Independently of all of these efforts, but focused on the same goals, Tadamitsu Kishimoto's group developed bioassays for human B cell Ig production from B cell lymphomas as well as B blast cells isolated from Staphylococcal-A-activated human tonsil cells in 1985.[44] As a source of T cell-derived factors, they established a human T leukemia cell line that spontaneously released an activity that promoted Ig production. Toshio Hirano identified proteins of 19 and 21 kDa (Mr), which he purified to homogeneity using several preparative steps, assaying relative concentrations using the reciprocal of the dilution that yielded 50% maximal Ig production as in the TCGF bioassay.[44] In 1986, cDNA probes were constructed based on amino acid sequences of the purified proteins, and used to identify clones from a cDNA library from the leukemic T cells that encoded a novel protein of 212 amino acid residues with 28 hydrophobic residues in the N-terminus.[45] Thus, the mature protein consisted of 184 amino acids and a calculated $M_r = 20,782$. Of the known cytokine sequences, only human G-CSF showed significant homology. Tests of biological activity of the purified protein indicated that this new cytokine promoted Ig production by both normal and malignant human B cells, but did not promote B cell proliferation.[46] Subsequently, this molecule became known as IL-6.

Thus, more than 15 years after the first descriptions of macrophage and T cell-derived activities found to "help" AFC formation and Ig production, three new interleukin molecules had been defined, isolated, characterized and sequenced. Critical in this process were the development of new assays that were amenable to quantitative analysis like the IL-2 bioassay. However, despite this progress, none of the new interleukin molecules, either alone or in combination, could effectively promote long-term B cell proliferation and cloning as had been so successful using IL-2 to create T cell lines and clones. Accordingly, there seemed to be something missing, or different about activation and proliferation of B cells compared with T cells.

"Linked Recognition"

Looking back to Mitchison's 1971 "linked recognition",[15] the observation that T cells contributed some vital physical signal to B cells independently of soluble helper molecules had never been fully explained. Thus, a 1986 report from Edward Clark and Jeffery Ledbetter of a MoAb that recognized a 50kDa (M_r) surface molecule restricted to normal and neoplastic B cells was of interest, in that this MoAb augmented the proliferation of anti-IgM-activated human tonsil B cells.[47] This B cell surface molecule was subsequently given a classification of CD40, and Jacques Blanchereau's group then demonstrated the first long-term growth of human B cell lines using IL-4 and anti-CD40 in 1991.[48] Because it had been shown that resting T cells proliferate to anti-CD3 bound to mouse fibroblastic cells expressing FcγRII, several MoAbs reactive with various B cell surface molecules were tested with these FcR+ cells for their capacity to activate the proliferation of highly purified resting human B cells. Only MoAbs reactive with CD40 induced proliferation. Particularly noteworthy, addition of recombinant IL-4 strongly enhanced the B cell proliferation, whereas the addition of IL-2 only weakly enhanced proliferation. B cells could be cultured with this combination for up to 10 weeks, and could be cloned by limiting dilution using the anti-CD40 MoAb bound to the FcγRII-expressing cells + IL-4.

Then within the span of a year, in 1992 four groups reported finding a surface molecule expressed by mitogen-activated Th cells that bound to B cell CD40 and activated both their proliferation and differentiation to AFCs. Seth Lederman working in Leonard Chess's group found that a clone of the human T leukemia cell line JURKAT possessed the unique capacity to induce the expression of B cell CD23. Using this clone, a MoAb was generated that bound to the T cell clone and inhibited activated T cells from inducing B cell CD23 expression.[49,50] Similarly, Melanie Spriggs' group found that human CD40 bound to the murine thymoma cell line, EL4. Using an expression cDNA library constructed from EL4 mRNA and biotinylated CD40, a cDNA was cloned that encoded a 260-amino acid residue protein with a calculated M_r = 29,395, which they termed CD40-ligand (CD40L). cDNA transfected paraformaldehyde-fixed cells activated the proliferation of murine splenic B cells and the addition of IL-4 promoted their production of IgE. In addition, Randolph Noelle's group had already reported that paraformaldehyde-fixed mitogen-activated Th cells and their purified plasma membranes induced B cell cycle entry and that IL-4, but not IL-2, IL-5 or IFNγ, augmented B cell DNA synthesis.[51] Using a human CD40-Ig fusion protein, they identified a 39 kDa surface molecule on activated but not resting Th cells, and raised a MoAb that reacted with this protein that blocked the induction of B cell cycle entry.[52] Finally, two separate groups isolated human cDNA clones encoding the human homologue of the murine CD40-L.[53,54]

The power of this molecular and genetic insight thus gained was immediately realized by 1993 reports from three groups and a total of 10 individuals who suffered from X-linked hyper-IgM syndrome, which is a rare genetic disorder characterized by normal or elevated levels of serum IgM but undetectable levels of IgG, IgA, and IgE.[55–57] Circulating B cell concentrations were normal, but the cells exclusively expressed only surface IgM/IgD. Affected males are unusually susceptible to recurrent pyogenic infections, autoimmune diseases, and lymphoproliferative diseases, thus a curious paradoxical mixture of immunodeficiency and autoimmunity, very similar to Miller's neonatal thymectomized mice first described >30 years earlier.[58] Genetic mapping of the CD40-L gene revealed that it is located in the q26.3–q27.1 region of the X chromosome,[54] while X-linked hyper-IgM syndrome had previously been assigned to Xq26. Various genetic mutations in the 10 individuals accounted for either the total lack of CD40-L expression, or to expression of CD40-L protein that failed to bind CD40. Accordingly, these reports solidified the only non-redundant function of the CD40-L/CD40 interaction is the important Ig class switch recombination that governs the switch from the μ-constant region to the other constant region H-chain isotypes.

The molecular explanation of T cell help of B cell proliferation and differentiation to AFCs, as residing in both soluble interleukin molecules and cell surface ligand/receptor pairs, yielded á new understanding of how messages are passed between the cells comprising the immune system. The unraveling of the various new interleukin molecules involved in T cell help was long and laborious but was ultimately successful because of the use of cloned T cells and the creation of quantitative bioassays, amenable to biochemical and genetic analysis of the various activities. The initial results of these advances immediately became apparent in new understanding of genetic mutations responsible for primary immunodeficiencies. Thus, the pathways were opened to a further molecular delineation, dissection, and elucidation of the TCR complex, the various interleukin receptors, the biochemical signaling pathways and genes activated by these newly discovered adaptive immune molecules.

References

1. Tees R and Schreier M. (1980). Selective reconstitution of nude mice with long-term cultured and cloned specific helper cells. *Nature* **283**:780–781.
2. Schreier M, Iscove N, Tees R, *et al.* (1980). Clones of killer and helper T cells: Growth requirements, specificity and retention of function in long-term culture. *Immunol Rev* **51**:315–336.
3. Hapel A, Lee J, Farrar W and Ihle J. (1981). Establishment of continuous cultures of Thy1.2+, Lyt1+, 2- T cells with purified interleukin-3. *Cell* **25**:179–186.
4. Ledbetter J, Rouse R, Micklem, H and Herzenberg L. (1980). T cell subsets defined by expression of Lyt1,2,3 and Thy1 antigens. Two parameter immunofluorescence and cytotoxicity analysis with monoclonal antibodies modifies current views. *J Exp Med* **152**:280.
5. Reinherz EL, Kung PC, Goldstein G and Schlossman SF. (1979). Separation of functional subsets of human T cells by a monoclonal antibody. *Proc Natl Acad Sci USA* **76**:4061–4065.

6. Weinstein Y. (1977). Twenty-alpha-hydroxysteroid dehydrogenase: A T lymphocyte-associated enzyme. *J Immunol* **119**:1223–1228.

7. Ihle J, Pepersack L, and Rebar L. (1981). Regulation of T cell differentiation: *in vitro* induction of 20alpha-hydroxysteroid dehydrogenase in splenic lymphocytes from athymic mice by a unique lymphokine. *J Immunol* **126**:2184–2189.

8. Schrader J. (1981). The *in vitro* production and cloning of the P cell, a bone marrow-derived null cell that expresses H-2 and Ia antigens, has mast cell-like granules, and is regulated by a factor released by activated T cells. *J Immunol* **126**:452–458.

9. Schrader J, Lewis S, Clark-Lewis I and Culvenor J. (1981). The persisting cell: Histamine content, regulation by a T cell-derived factor, origin from a bone marrow precursor, and relationship to mast cells. *Proc Natl Acad Sci USA* **78**:323–327.

10. Schrader J and Clark-Lewis I. (1982). A T cell-derived factor stimulating multipotential hematopoietic stem cells: Molecular weight and distinction from T cell growth factor and T cell-derived granulocyte-macrophage colony-stimulating factor. *J Immunol* **129**:30–35.

11. Fung M, Hapel A, Ymer S, *et al.* (1984). Molecular cloning of cDNA for murine interleukin-3. *Nature* **307**:233–237.

12. Smith KA, Favata MF and Oroszlan S. (1983). Production and characterization of monoclonal antibodies to human interleukin 2: Strategy and tactics. *J Immunol* **131**:1808–1815.

13. Taniguchi T, Matsui H, Fujita T, *et al.* (1983). Structure and expression of a cloned cDNA for human interleukin-2. *Nature* **302**:305–310.

14. Hapel A, Fung M, Johnson R, *et al.* (1985). Biological properties of molecularly cloned and expressed murine interleukin-3. *Blood* **65**:1453–1459.

15. Mitchison N. (1971). The carrier effect in the secondary response to hapten-protein conjugates. II Cellular cooperation. *Euro J Immunol* **1**:18–27.

16. Hoffman M and Dutton R. (1971). Immune response restoration with macrophage culture supernatants. *Science* **172**:1047–1048.

17. Schimpl A and Wecker E. (1972). Replacement of T cell function by a T cell product. *Nature New Biol.* **237**:15–17.

18. Baker PE, Gillis S and Smith KA. (1979). Monoclonal cytolytic T-cell lines. *J Exp Med* **149**:273–278.

19. Jerne NK, and Nordin AA. (1963). Antibody formation in agar by single antibody-producing cells. *Science* **140**:405.

20. Mishell R and Dutton R. (1967). Immunization of dissociated spleen cell cultures from normal mice. *J Exp Med* **126**:423–442.

21. Andersson J, Schreier M and Melchers F. (1980). T-cell-dependent B-cell stimulationis H-2-restricted and antigen-dependent only at the resting B-cell level. *Proc Natl Acad Sci USA* **77**:1612–1616.

22. Melchers F, Andersson J, Lernhardt W and Schreier M. (1980). H-2-unrestricted polyclonal maturation without replication of small B cells induced by antigen-activated T cell helper factors. *Eur J Immunol* **10**:679–685.

23. Andersson J, Moller G and Sjoberg O. (1972). Selective induction of DNA synthesis in T and B lymphocytes. *Cell Immunol* **4**:381–393.

24. Schreier M and Iscove N. (1980). Hematopoietic growth factors are released in cultures of H-2-restricted helper T cells, accessory cells and specific antigen. *Nature* **287**:228–230.

25. Pure E, Isakson P, Takatsu K, *et al.* (1981). Induction of B cell differentiation by T cell factors. I. Stimulation of IgM secretion by products of a T cell hybridoma and a T cell line. *J Immunol* **127**:1953–1958.

26. Swain S, Dennert G, Warner J and Dutton R. (1981). Culture supernatants of a stimulated T-cell line have helper activity that acts synergistically with interleukin-2 in the response of B cells to antigen. *Proc Natl Acad Sci USA* **78**:2517–2521.

27. Isakson P, Pure E, Vitteta E and Krammer P. (1982). T cell-derived B cell differentiation factor(s): Effect on the isotype switch of murine B cells. *J Exp Med* **155**:734–748.

28. Howard M, Farrar J, Hilfiker M, *et al.* (1982). Identification of a T cell-derived B cell growth factor distinct from interleukin 2. *J Exp Med* **155**:914–923.

29. Parker D. (1980). Induction and suppression of polyclonal antibody responses by anti-Ig reagents and antigen-nonspecific helper factors. *Immunol Rev* **52**:115–135.

30. Cantrell DA and Smith KA. (1984). The interleukin-2 T-cell system: A new cell growth model. *Science* **224**:1312–1316.

31. Smith KA. (1980). T-cell growth factor. *Immunol Rev* **51**:337–357.

32. Howard M, Mizel S, Lachman L, *et al.* Role of interleukin-1 in anti-immunoglobulin induced B cell proliferation. *J Exp Med* **157**:1529–1543.

33. Smith KA, Gilbride KJ and Favata MF. (1980). Lymphocyte activating factor promotes T-cell growth factor production by cloned murine lymphoma cells. *Nature* **287**:853–855.

34. Smith KA, Lachman LB, Oppenheim JJ, and Favata MF. (1980). The functional relationship of the interleukins. *J Exp Med* **151**:1551–1556.

35. Swain S, Howard M, Kappler J, et al. (1983). Evidence for two distinct classes of murine B cell growth factors with activities in different functional assays. *J Exp Med* **158**:822–835.

36. Howard M, Matis L, Malek T, et al. (1983). Interleukin-2 induces antigen-reactive T cell lines to secrete BCGF-I. *J Exp Med* **158**:2024–2039.

37. Sideras P, Bergstedt-Lindqvist S, MacDonald H, and Severinson E. (1985). Secretion of IgG1 induction factor by T cell clones and hybridomas. *Eur J Immunol* **15**:586–593.

38. Ohara J and Paul W. (1985). Production of a monoclonal antibody to and molecular characterization of B cell stimulatory factor-1. *Nature* **315**:333–336.

39. Sideras P, Bergstedt-Lindqvist S and Severinson E. (1985). Partial biochemical characterization of IgG-inducing factor. *Eur J Immunol* **15**:593–598.

40. Noma Y, Sideras P, Naito T, et al. (1986). Cloning of cDNA encoding the murine IgG1 induction factor by a novel strategy using SP6 promoter. *Nature* **319**:640–646.

41. Lee F, Yokota T, Otsuka T, et al. (1986). Isolation and chracterization of a mouse interleukin cDNA clone that expresses B cellstimulatory factor-1 activities and T cell- and mast cell-stimulating activities. *Proc Natl Acad Sci USA* **83**:2061–2065.

42. Sanderson C, O'Garra A, Warren D and Klaus G. (1986). Eosinophil differentiation factor also has B cell growth factor activity: Proposed name interleukin-4. *Proc Natl Acad Sci USA* **83**:437–440.

43. Kinashi T, Harada N, Severinson E, et al. (1986). Cloning of complementary DNA encoding T cell replacing factor and identity with B cell growth factor II. *Nature* **324**:70–73.

44. Hirano T, Taga T, Kakano N, et al. (1985). Purification to homogeneity and chracterization of human B cell differentiation factor (BCDF or BSFp-2). *Proc Natl Acad Sci USA* **82**:5490–5494.

45. Hirano T, Yasukawa K, Harada H, et al. (1986). Complementary DNA for a novel human interleukin (BSF-2) that induces B lymphocytes to produce immunoglobulin. *Nature* **324**:73–76.

46. Hirano T, Taga T, Nakano N, et al. (1985). Purification to homogeneity and characterization of human B-cell differentiation factor (BCDF or BSFp-2). *Proc Natl Acad Sci USA* **82**:5490–5494.

47. Clark E and Ledbetter J. (1986). Activation of human B cells mediated through two distinct cell surface differentiation antigens, Bp35 and Bp50. *Proc Natl Acad Sci USA* **83**:4494–4498.

48. Blanchereau J, De Pauli P, Valle A, et al. (1991). Long-term human B cell lines dependent on interleukin-4 and antibody to CD40. Science 251:70–72.

49. Lederman S, Yellin M, Krichevsky A, et al. (1992). Identification of a novel surface protein on activated CD4+ T cells that induces contact-dependent B cell differentiation (help). J Exp Med 175:1091–1099.

50. Lederman S, Yellin MJ, Inghirami G, et al. (1992). Molecular interactions mediating T-B lymphocyte collaboration in human lymphoid follicles. Roles of T cell-B cell activating molecules (5c8 antigen) and CD40 in contact-dependent help. J Immunol 149:3817–3826.

51. Bartlett W, McCann J, Shepherd D, et al. (1990). Cognate interactions between helper T cells and B cells. IV. Requirements for the expression of effector phase activity by helper T cells. J Immunol 145:3956–3962.

52. Noelle R, Roy M, Shepherd D, et al. (1992). A 39-kDa protein on activated helper T cells binds CD40 and transduces the signal for cognate activation of B cells. Proc Natl Acad Sci USA 89:6550–6554.

53. Spriggs M, Armitage R, Strockbine L, et al. (1992). Recombinant human CD40 ligand stimulates B cell proliferation and immunoglobulin E secretion. J Exp Med 176:1543–1550.

54. Graf D, Korthauer G, Mages H, et al. (1992). Cloning of TRAP, a ligand for CD40 on human T cells. Eur. J Immunol 22:3191–3194.

55. Korthauer U, Graf D, Mages H, et al. (1993). Defective expression of T-cell CD40 ligand causes X-linked immunodeficiency with hyper IgM. Nature 361:539–541.

56. DiSanto J, Bonnefoy J, Gauchat J, et al. (1993). CD40 ligand mutations in X-linked hyper IgM. Nature 361:341–343.

57. Fuleihan R, Ramesh N, Loh R, et al. (1993). Defective expression of the CD40 ligand in X chromosome-linked immunoglobulin deficiency with normal or elevated IgM. Proc Natl Acad Sci USA 90:2170–2173.

58. Miller J. (1962). Effect of neonatal thymectomy on the immunological responsiveness of the mouse. Proc Roy Soc London-B 156:415–428.

6 The Molecules of Macrophages

Macrophages: Essential for Adaptive Immunity

From the days of Eli Metchnikoff's original descriptions of phagocytosis by starfish larvae, which he observed via light microscopy in the late 19th century, macrophages and the process of phagocytosis gripped investigators who followed his lead in the idea that phagocytic cells ultimately mediated immunity.[1] However, as the 20th century moved on, another school stemmed from the 1890 report by Emil von Behring and Shibasaburo Kitasato[2] that blood sera contains an antibacterial substance that protects animals from both diphtheria and tetanus. Thus, the idea that humoral factors might be responsible for immunity took hold, and eventually eclipsed the importance of cellular immunity mediated by macrophages among the immunology cognoscenti. In this regard, Astrid Fagraeus had shown by 1948 that after the injection of an antigen, plasma cells appear in the spleen coincident with circulating antibody activity.[3] Even so, at the time it was not at all appreciated that lymphocytes are the precursors to the antibody-forming plasma cells (AFC). For example, Fagraeus speculated that reticulo-endothelial cells were perhaps the source of plasma cells, and stated that she found no evidence that lymphocytes participated in their generation.[3] Furthermore, Neils Jerne's 1955 hypothesis of the natural selection of antibody formation[4] was based on the idea that antigen-antibody complexes engulfed by phagocytes were used as intracellular molecular templates so that additional antibodies could be selected and synthesized by the phagocytic cells.

Burnet first hypothesized, and published, that lymphocytes and not macrophages were the precursors of AFCs in 1957.[5] Then in 1963

Jerne demonstrated that lymphoid cells were found at the center of the *in vitro* hemolytic antibody plaques formed from splenocytes taken from rabbits and mice immunized with sheep red blood cells (RBCs).[6] Subsequently, as detailed in Chapter 1,[7] with the advent of the capacity to generate the formation of antibody-forming cells (AFC) *in vitro* via the Mishell Dutton system,[8] Donald Mosier revealed that macrophages are an essential cell in the murine splenocyte populations used to enumerate AFCs.[9] Thus, although lymphoid cells were the AFC precursors, removal of the macrophages abrogated the generation of AFCs.

If macrophages were not the source of plasma cells and antibodies, but were required for the generation of AFCs from lymphoid cells, the question became what role these phagocytic cells played in adaptive immunity. Phagocytosis from the time of Metchnikoff had been studied using particulate matter, such as bacteria, and the light microscope, which magnified objects maximally 400–1000-fold (attributed to a 10× ocular and 40× and 100× objective lenses). Barbara Ehrenreich and Zanvil Cohn first studied the phagocytic process in 1967 using radioiodinated human serum albumin (HSA) as a small protein molecule together with autoradiography. They found that radioiodinated HSA was taken up by murine macrophages through pinocytosis, trafficked to lysosomes, degraded into monoiodotyrosine and excreted from the cells with a half-time ($t^{1/2}$) of ~ five hours.[10] With this efficient digestion of antigenic molecules, one wondered how antigens were retained long enough to promote lymphoid cells to produce antibody molecules.

Subsequently in 1968, Emil Unanue and Brigitte Askonas studied the uptake, catabolism, persistence, and immunogenicity of radiolabeled antigen in macrophages, which allowed them to quantify accurately the degradation process.[11] When murine macrophages were cultured with radioiodinated hemocyanin, the cells rapidly catabolized most of the antigen, but ~10% of the iodinated antigen was retained by the cells for up to two days. By transfer of the live macrophages containing this small amount of radiolabeled antigen to syngeneic hosts, these investigators found retention of immunogenicity for up to two weeks. Accordingly, there appeared to be some mechanism whereby macrophages held on to a small amount of the antigen in a form protected from rapid breakdown and elimination, and this cell-associated form somehow promoted the generation of specific antibodies.

Using electron micrographic (EM) autoradiography (magnification × 11,700) with radioiodinated hemocyanin, Unanue went on to show in 1969 that after the initial digestion of antigenic molecules, ~20% of the labeled molecules could be localized to the cell periphery, on or just contiguous with the cell membrane, or in small villous projections of the macrophage surface.[12] Also, the surface radiolabel was sensitive to protease trypsin, but was insensitive to ribonuclease or neuraminidase. Since the hemocyanin molecules were huge, >10^6 Da, and because hemocyanin-reactive antibodies also reacted with the surface of antigen-pulsed macrophages, it was interpreted that the hemocyanin molecules on the surface of the macrophages were intact, and somehow had escaped the intracellular digestive process. In a separate 1970 publication, Unanue and Cerottini further stated that: "*It is apparent that the plasma membrane is a site where some molecules of antigen escape degradation and can, therefore, retain their original structure. Hence, the antibody response to macrophage-bound antigen may still be directed to conformational determinants of the native antigen.*"[13]

Macrophage Soluble Products as Lymphocyte Activating Factors (LAF) and Endogenous Pyrogens (EP)

After the original 1965 descriptions of "Blastogenic Factor" found in the culture supernatants of mixed leukocyte cultures,[14–16] Fritz Bach's team first described a macrophage-derived soluble factor that potentiated lymphocyte proliferative responses in 1970,[16] and Michael Hoffman and Richard Dutton described a soluble macrophage activity that could replace the macrophage requirement for the *in vitro* generation of AFCs in 1971.[17] Subsequently in 1972, Igal Gery, working with Byron Waksman confirmed Joost Oppenheim's 1968 report,[18] that lymphocytes depleted of glass-adherent cells proliferated poorly in response to mitogenic lectins,[19] and then went on to show that adherent cells produce a soluble activity, especially when cultured with bacterial endotoxin, lipopolysaccharide (LPS), that potentiated the mitogenic response of purified thymocyte or peripheral lymphocytes.[20] They named this activity Lymphocyte Activating Factor (LAF). Similar findings were reported in 1972 by my lab-mate Leonard Chess, who showed that synthetic polyribonucleotides, such as polyadenylic acid and polyuridylic acid (polyA:U), augmented the specific antigen-induced proliferative response of human peripheral blood mononuclear cells (PBMCs), and that this activity could be localized to an effect on plastic-adherent cells.[21] Synthetic polyribonucleotides had already been shown in 1971 by John Schmidke and Arthur Johnson to be potent immunological adjuvants in experimental animals *in vivo*,[22] and subsequently in 1976 by my laboratory to also induce both fever and interferon production in humans *in vivo*.[23] Thus, in addition to their phagocytic activity and their apparent capacity to present immunogenic proteins on their cell surface, macrophages were found to produce soluble activities that potentiated antigen-specific lymphocyte proliferation *in vitro*, and macrophage stimulants such as LPS and polyribonucleotides possessed adjuvant activity *in vivo*. Even so, without molecular characterization, it was impossible to ascertain whether only one or several molecules were responsible for these various activities. Moreover, it was unclear as to whether the macrophage stimulants, LPS and ployribonucleotides, or the macrophage products accounted for the adjuvant activity.

A separate, but related line of investigation evolved from physicians interested in understanding the molecular basis of fever. From the original 1953 descriptions of Ivan Bennett and Paul Beeson, it had been established that polymorphonuclear (PMN) phagocytes (termed *microphages* by Metchnikoff) contained heat labile, nondialyzable substances that caused fever when injected into rabbits.[24] Subsequently, the identification of patients with agranulocytosis and fever alerted investigators to the possibility that other cells, in addition to PMNs, might be sources of what came to be termed endogenous pyrogens (EP). Thus, in 1967 Phyllis Bodel and Elisha Atkins first described that blood monocytes are capable of releasing an EP after stimulation via phagocytosis of heat-killed Staphylococci.[25] In 1974,

Charles Dinarello working in Sheldon Wolff's group, first reported detailed biochemical analyses of EPs from both PMNs and monocytes.[26] Following incubation with heat-killed Staphylococci, monocyte preparations contained 20-times more pyrogenic activity than did an equal number of PMNs, as monitored by fever production in rabbits. Moreover, the two pyrogens could be distinguished on gel filtration, with the monocyte pyrogen migrating at ~38 kDa, while the PMN pyrogen migrated at ~15 kDa.

MHC Restriction of Antigen Recognition: Antigen Presentation

As detailed in Chapter 1, Baruj Benacerraf and his group first showed that synthetic polypeptides could elicit delayed type hypersensitivity (DTH) responses in 1963.[27] Also, a short time later Stuart Schlossman, investigating the types of antigens capable of eliciting both immediate and DTH responses, reported in 1966 that a minimum of eight amino acid residues were required for polypeptides to generate a DTH response.[28] Concomitantly, Benacerraf's team showed that immune responsiveness to short synthetic peptides in guinea pigs was genetically linked, and that there were high and low responders.[29] Then, in 1968 when Hugh McDevitt's team first found the genetic regulation of the antibody response to synthetic peptides was linked to the Major Histocompatibility Complex (MHC),[30] the notion that antigen presenting cells (APC) somehow were involved in immune regulation began to take shape. In 1973, Alan Rosenthal and Ethan Shevach first reported a requirement for histocompatibility between T cells and macrophages for an antigen-specific T cell proliferative response,[31] and Benacerraf's group showed that B cells and T cells must share MHC genes for the generation of antigen-specific AFCs.[32]

Also, humoral immune responses were known by this time to require at least three cell types, B cells, macrophages and T cells. However, understanding of the molecular basis of genetic restriction was hampered by the lack of a molecular characterization of the MHC gene products that were termed Immune response (Ir) gene products, or immune-associated (Ia) molecules, as it had not been possible to generate antisera reactive with them: instead, they were defined by mixed lymphocyte culture (MLC) reactivity. Now, these are known as MHC Class II gene-encoded molecules.

A significant advance occurred when Rolf Zinkernagel and Peter Doherty reported in 1974 that cytotoxic T cells were also restricted by MHC gene products, but in this case the T cells and the target cells had to share the serologically defined MHC encoded molecules, now known to be encoded by Class I MHC genes.[33] Much excitement as well as confusion followed until Baruj Benacerraf clarified the issue considerably in 1978 by hypothesizing that "*the Ir gene products on macrophages and B cells interact specifically with unique amino acid sequences of the antigen concerned*", and that these peptides were then recognized by specific T cells responsible for providing "help" for AFC generation and for DTH.[34] Benacerraf went on to say, "*Intentionally, this theory does not concern the nature of the T cell receptors or receptors, nor the possibility that there could be more than one T cell receptor as proposed by some investigators, one for the antigen and the other for the Ia molecule, since both possibilities are totally compatible with the present hypothesis.*"[34] He also postulated that his hypothesis could be extended to explain the genetic restriction of the CTL/target cell interactions, such that the MHC encoded Class I molecules could also bind specific amino acid determinants derived from antigenic peptides. It's of more than passing interest that this hypothesis essentially clinched the Nobel Prize for Benacerraf, which he shared with George Snell and Jean Dausset in 1980 for their collective work in the discovery and functional importance of the MHC genes for the immune response.

Lymphocyte Activation: Soluble "Factors"

Since the original descriptions of the macrophage-derived LAFs in the early 1970s, considerable confusion evolved regarding the roles of macrophage soluble activities in lymphocyte activation. Thus, as stated in 1979 by several investigators working in the field, "*in addition to their role of "presenting" antigen to T cells in association with surface membrane components such as Ia, macrophages release a battery of soluble factors that stimulate proliferation and differentiation of lymphoid cells.*"[35] Because the number and characteristics of the molecules responsible for the soluble activities had yet to be elucidated, it was impossible to ascertain the relative contributions of these macrophage functions in lymphocyte activation. It is noteworthy that most of these investigators worked with murine cells and soluble LAFs.

Emil Unanue examined murine peritoneal exudate cells and reported that various agents added to the cells *in vitro,* including latex particles, antibody-coated red cells, endotoxin, Listeria bacteria, or beryllium salts, increased the production of soluble activities mitogenic for murine thymocytes.[36] Also, the addition of T cells from Listeria-infected mice increased the putative macrophage-derived activities a great deal. Thus, the idea that perhaps there was a cyclical interaction between macrophages and T cells mediated via soluble molecules was introduced: soluble macrophage activities enhanced the release of T cell-derived activities, which then enhanced the release of more macrophage activities, etc.

By 1977 Charles Dinarello focusing on characterizing human EP, had successfully generated rabbit antisera that neutralized EP activity in the rabbit fever bioassay.[37] To produce EP, human PBMCs were mixed with heat-killed Staphylococci as a phagocytic stimulus in media with 10% human sera for 30 minutes, then washed and cultured sera-free for 18 hours. The crude culture supernatants were then harvested, concentrated, and used for immunizations. The EP neutralizing activity in the sera from immunized animals was found in the Ig fractions, and was specific for human EP, being nonreactive with guinea pig, monkey and rabbit EP, all of which scored positive in the rabbit fever bioassay. Furthermore, solid-phase immunoadsorbant columns constructed with the antisera could be used to concentrate EP bioactivity ~50-fold. Even so, biochemical analysis of the eluted immunoadsorbed EP indicated that it was by no means a homogeneous single protein molecule, but the bioactivity could be localized to a 15kDa moiety among the several proteins eluted.

Concomitantly, in 1977 Monte Meltzer and Joost Oppenheim examined murine adherent peritoneal cells for their capacity to produce LAF, and in the process developed a LAF assay, based on Igal

Gery's seminal 1972 studies[19] using murine thymocytes, which subsequently became standard to monitor LAF activity.[38] Thymocytes · from C57Bl/6, C3H/HeJ or BC3F$_1$ 6–8-week-old mice were suspended at a high density (7.5 × 10^6 cells/mL) in culture medium with 5% FCS together with dilutions of macrophage supernatants, and cultured for 3-days. Cultures were pulsed for the final 4–5 hours of the culture period with tritiated thymidine (^{3}H-TdR), then harvested and counted in a liquid scintillation counter. Preliminary experiments showed undetectable activity at dilutions 1/8 or greater of the supernatants so that ¼ dilutions were used solely thereafter and absolute CPMs were monitored in triplicate. A representative experiment yielded 200 ± 30 CPM from supernatants of adherent peritoneal cells cultured for 3-days with medium alone, and 1480 ± 10 CPM from supernatants of cell aliquots cultured with 50 µg/mL LPS for 3-days. Accordingly, a very high thymocyte cell density yielded only very low ^{3}H-TdR incorporation, with a Simulation Index (SI) of only ~7-fold. This assay relied upon a "direct" mitogenic effect of the adherent cell supernatants. However, it was also shown that a submitogenic concentration of PHA (1µg/mL) augmented the thymocyte ^{3}H-TdR incorporation, thereby increasing the signal-noise ratio.

Meltzer and Oppenheim also introduced LAF produced by a macrophage-like cell line, P388D$_1$ which originated as a methylcholantrene-induced lymphoid neoplasm from a DBA/2 mouse (P388). After ~50 passages *in vivo,* a "derived" culture line (P388D$_1$) was initiated in August, 1956, and carried *in vitro* continuously by C. J. Dawe and W. D. Morgan at the National Cancer Institute.[39] In 1975, John Wunderlich and co-workers characterized this cell line after its 179th *in vitro* passage, finding that it expressed most, if not all, of the normal characteristics of macrophages.[39] Then, in 1977 Meltzer and Oppenheim found that P388D$_1$ cells produced ~10-fold greater amounts of LAF activity compared with normal macrophages when stimulated by LPS. In addition to these data confirming Unanue's findings, they also reported that antigen-induced splenocytes produced a "lymphokine" activity that augmented LAF production by both normal macrophages and P388D$_1$ cells.[38] In other 1977 experiments, Lawrence Lachman working with Robert

Handschumacher then extended these observations, reporting that in addition to P388D$_1$, the murine macrophage-like cell lines J774, WEHI-3, and PU5-1.8 also produced LAF activity in serum-free medium after stimulation with LPS, as monitored by the thymocyte assay.[40] Biochemical analysis revealed that the LAF activity had an apparent molecular size of 75–80 KDa, whereas human LAF activity, derived from normal human monocytes was found at 12–13 KDa.

By 1978, the year that Benacerraf hypothesized that MHC encoded molecules functioned to "present" antigenic peptides to responding T cells, Steven Mizel working in Oppenheim's group, focused on the biological and biochemical characteristics of LAF activity produced by P388D$_1$ cells induced by both activated T cells and LPS in only 1% FCS.[41,42] Activities were monitored using a single supernatant concentration (1/4 dilution) and the thymocyte assay with and without submitogenic concentrations of PHA (1 µg/mL). They reported that mouse and guinea pig T cells activated with PHA "*produced very little LAF activity*", but when the T cells were co-cultured with the P388D$_1$ cells, there was a marked enhancement of LAF activity compared with simply the P388D$_1$ cells alone pulsed with PHA. Biochemical analysis yielded results indicating that both T cell-stimulated and LPS-stimulated P388D$_1$ LAF activity had similar molecular sizes (~16 KDa) as monitored by molecular gel filtration, and charges as monitored by ion exchange chromatography. Moreover, analysis of LAF activity from normal murine macrophages yielded similar results, so that these investigators concluded that the P388D$_1$-dervied supernatants could be used for further biochemical characterizations[42].

From all of these experiments performed by several groups it was clear that the biochemical analyses revealed that several distinct molecules might well contribute LAF activity. However, it was difficult to proceed with further analyses despite the identification of P388D$_1$ as a homogeneous cell source for the activities, in that the thymocyte assay utilized a heterogeneous target cell population for the detection of LAF activity. Furthermore, it was not clear why such a high thymocyte cell density was required, nor why more mitogenic activity was found when a submitogenic concentration of PHA or

ConA was present in the assay. Finally, the relationship of LPS-derived LAF and activated T cell-promoted LAF activity suggested a molecular complexity that would be difficult to dissect. As stated by Byron Waksman at the 2nd International Lymphokine Workshop held in 1979, "*One cannot help feeling that it is just as important to define the real* (cell) *target of the agent as the actual* (molecular) *agent. The use of whole thymocytes as an assay population is a particularly vivid example of this problem especially when one assays* ^{3}*H-TdR incorporation at 72 hours.*"[43]

A step in the right direction was reported by Lanny Rosenwasser, Charles Dinarello and Alan Rosenthal who collaborated in 1979 to explore whether LAF activity and EP activity could be similar or identical.[44] For their assay, instead of murine thymocytes they utilized macrophage-depleted murine lymph node cells (90–95% T cells, 1–5% B cells, 0.1–0.5% macrophages) from mice immunized with specific antigen (dinitrophenyl-egg albumin; DNP_{13}-OVA) to assay for LAF/EP activities. These investigators hypothesized that there were at least two functions for macrophages that supported antigen-specific T cell proliferative responses: macrophage-derived soluble factors that are neither antigen-specific nor MHC-restricted in their activities, and an antigen presenting function that is MHC-dependent and restricted, as reported originally by Rosenthal and Shevach using guinea pig cells.[31] Thus, they found that soluble macrophage-derived activities could partially (~50%) replace macrophage-dependent antigen-specific T cell proliferative responses, and most important, affinity-purified human EP functioned equally as well as murine macrophage-derived LAF activity. Thus, they speculated that "*some, if not all, LAF-like activity is due to EP.*"[44] Perhaps of even greater significance for EP, this finding indicated that a murine T cell *in vitro* proliferative LAF-like bioassay could replace the much more cumbersome and time-consuming *in vivo* rabbit fever bioassay.

The Interleukins

Obviously, the field suffered from heterogeneity, i.e. heterogeneity of cells producing the factor activities, heterogeneity of molecules responsible for the activities, and heterogeneity of bioassay target cells. A breakthrough occurred in 1977 with the creation of antigen-specific cytotoxic T lymphocyte lines (CTLL)[45] and especially CTL clones, the asexual progeny of a single cell,[46] in that for the first time the target cell heterogeneity was solved. The story of the scientific rationale behind the interleukin nomenclature was told in Chapter 1, so that it would be redundant to recount it here. However, from the viewpoint of macrophages, the surprise to everyone in the field was the finding that preparations that had LAF activity in the thymocyte and macrophage-depleted T cell proliferation assays had no activity in the CTLL T-cell Growth Factor (TCGF) assay, when CTL lines or clones were used as target cells. By comparison, in 1980 we found that preparations with TCGF activity scored positive in the LAF assays.[47,48] Although T cells were the likely source of TCGF, its production was macrophage-dependent, similar to lectin/antigen-induced T cell proliferation.[47]

One logical hypothesis that would explain this dichotomy was that LAF from macrophages enhanced the production of TCGF by T cells. Moreover, it appeared that there were at least two types of T cells, TCGF-producer cells and TCGF responder cells, and that CTLL and clones must be TCGF responder but not producer cells.[47] Accordingly, we tested this hypothesis in 1980, and showed that cloned murine T lymphoma cells produced TCGF in a LAF concentration-dependent manner, using human LPS-stimulated LAF partially purified by gel filtration and isoelectric focusing.[49] Thus, we concluded that LAF and TCGF appeared to constitute "*a bimodal amplification system*," since TCGF production was dependent on the concentration of LAF available, and the rate and extent of T cell proliferation was TCGF concentration-dependent.[49] Similar findings and conclusions were reported by Eva Lotta Larsson, Norman Iscove and Antonio Coutinho who used LAF activity partially purified from WEHI-3 cells, another macrophage-like cell line.[50] Additional experiments indicated that both the LPS-stimulated production of LAF by macrophages and the lectin-stimulated production of TCGF by T cells was inhibited by immunosuppressive glucocorticoid hormones, but the action of TCGF to promote CTLL proliferation was only mildly impaired by glucocorticoids.[51] All of these data led to the conclusion that LAF acted *before* TCGF in the promotion of mitogen/antigen initiated T cell proliferation, thereby justifying the nomenclature of IL-1 for LAF and IL-2 for TCGF.[52] Even so, the new nomenclature was premature, in that neither activities, although distinguishable functionally, had been shown to be attributed to purified, distinct homogeneous molecules.

Defining IL-1 Molecules

In 1981, Steven and Diane Mizel developed a "super-induction protocol" using phorbol myristic acetate, cycloheximide and actinomycin-D to activate the production of LAF activity by P388D$_1$ cells in 24 hours in media containing 1%FCS.[53] Starting with ~5L of conditioned media, they reported the purification of 64 μg of LAF activity to "apparent homogeneity." They used the standard thymocyte proliferation assay and borrowing from the TCGF bioassay, they tested serial two-fold dilutions of samples, and defined as standard an EC$_{50}$ having a concentration of 10 Units/mL (dilution = 1:10). However, after several analytic separative procedures there remained three distinct charged species, so that it was not clear whether they had actually attained purification to homogeneity. Moreover, it was difficult to prove homogeneity with additional tests because only microgram quantities of protein remained after the purification steps, in that the yield of bioactivity was only 1–2%. In addition, this small amount of protein was insufficient for additional biological characterization steps.

Realizing that a new preparative approach to purification would be necessary, Mizel and co-workers developed heterologous antisera reactive with IL-1 in 1983.[54] A goat was immunized weekly for seven injections of 10–15 μg partially purified murine IL-1. After absorption with murine thymocytes, the hyperimmune serum inhibited LAF activity in the standard thymocyte assay, and the inhibitory activity could be localized to the IgG fraction of the serum. In addition, this antiserum inactivated human LAF activity derived from the U937 macrophage-like cell line. When used as an immunoprecipitant and as an immunoadsorbant, proteins containing LAF activity could be obtained, although unexplained micro-heterogeneity persisted so that the exact molecular properties (size and charge) of IL-1 remained obscure.

This anti-IL-1 serum was then used to identify a cDNA encoding murine IL-1 activity by Mizel in collaboration with Peter Lomedico's group in 1984.[55] Using 'superinduced' vs. uninduced $P388D_1$ cells, polyA+ mRNA was prepared and translated *in vitro* followed by immunoprecipitation with the goat anti-IL-1 serum. A ~33 KDa protein was identified, and following positive selection hybridization, translation and immunoprecipitation a cDNA clone was identified that contained a polyA tract and a 1701 bp insert. This cDNA clone was then used to probe for a second clone that contained the 5' end of the coding region. The predicted amino acid sequence of the two overlapping clones indicated 270 amino acids (~33 KDa), but surprisingly without a signal peptide. Also surprising was the finding that the carboxy-terminal end of the protein, only 156 amino acids (~18 kDa) contained biological IL-1 activity as detected in the murine thymocyte assay. Moreover, recombinant immunoaffinity-purified protein fragments of this smaller size were active in the thymocyte bioassay. Thus, it was concluded that IL-1 is initially translated as a precursor of ~33 KDa that is processed to form the mature active protein of ~18 kDa. To account for the microheterogeneity of both size and charge that was seen after multiple purification schemes, the authors stated, *"We suggest that one or more proteases released by the macrophage may be responsible for cleaving at a primary processing site. Subsequent proteolytic activity would generate 'ragged' amino-termini, thus providing an explanation for the size and charge microheterogeneity that is characteristic for IL-1."* From the data presented, it was clear that a cDNA encoding a molecule that was recognized by the anti-IL-1 serum had been cloned, but it was not clear whether this was the only molecule with IL-1 activity. Also, it remained to be determined how the precursor and mature protein exited the cell.

Concomitantly, Charles Dinarello used his human EP/IL-1-specific rabbit antiserum to approach the identification and isolation of human cDNA clones encoding IL-1 activity.[37] To monitor for IL-1 activity, Dinarello's group took advantage of a report by Jonathan Kaye, working in Charles Janeway's group, who generated a murine IL-2-dependent helper T (Th) cell clone (D10.G4.1) that recognized an epitope contained within conalbumin, the minor protein component of avian egg albumin. Using this Th clone as an immunogen, a clone-specific MoAb was generated that only recognized a surface determinant unique to this clone (later shown to be the TCR), and which was mitogenic for the T cell clone, *provided* a source of IL-1 was present.[56] Noteworthy was the fact that if conalbumin was used as antigen without APCs, the Th clone would not proliferate even when IL-1 was provided. Accordingly, these results confirmed earlier data, showing that IL-1 provided a signal in addition to TCR triggering that was necessary to induce the Th clone to produce IL-2 and then to subsequently proliferate. The clonotypic MoAb was thus very useful because the Th clone + the TCR MoAb served as an IL-1 bioassay that could be interpreted unambiguously, since no other cells or triggers were involved, with the caveat that IL-2 would also score positive in this assay.

To identify a human IL-1 cDNA, PBMCs were seeded into glass flasks, and the adherent cells were stimulated for 12 hours with LPS.[57] The cells were then harvested and lysed with 6 M guanididium thiocyanate, and the poly(A)+ RNA fraction was isolated. An identical RNA fraction was isolated from uninduced cells. Using these RNA preparations, reticulocyte lysates were used to translate radiolabeled proteins that were immunoprecipitated using the IL-1 antiserum. A ~35 kDa band was identified as specific for the LPS-induced but not the uninduced cells. To isolate IL-1 cDNA, radiolabeled cDNA probes from LPS-induced and uninduced poly(A)+ RNA were used to differentially screen cDNA libraries constructed from LPS-induced poly(A)+ RNA. cDNA candidate clones were then used to hybrid select poly(A)+ RNA that was *in vitro* translated followed by immunoprecipitation. One clone was selected (~960 bp) and used as a probe to analyze mRNA from LPS-induced cells, which identified a single transcript of ~1,600 bp. A single cDNA clone of ~1,560 bp was then identified, and used to hybrid select poly(A)+ RNA that was injected into Xenopus laevis oocytes that secreted biologically active IL-1 activity as detected by the D10 T cell clone IL-1 bioassay. Accordingly, the putative human IL-1 cDNA clones ultimately identified encoded a protein of ~ 30 kDa that was immunoreactive as well as biologically reactive. The nucleotide sequence predicted a protein of 269 amino acids, which like the murine cDNA did not contain a hydrophobic amino-terminal signal peptide. Thus, in 1984 Dinarello's group interpreted their results as *"entirely possible that the extracellular appearance of IL-1 from stimulated monocytes is predominantly the result of cell "leakage" rather than active transport."*[57]

The following year 1985, Carl March and co-workers reported two distinct but distantly related human cDNAs encoding IL-1 activity.[58] To monitor IL-1 activity, an assay employing a murine lymphoma cell line that produced IL-2 in response to a combination of PHA and IL-1 was utilized.[59] This assay purportedly corresponded to the mouse thymocyte assay for IL-1, but was alleged to be 1,000-fold more sensitive. Poly(A)$^+$ RNA from LPS-induced human monocytes was selected to construct a cDNA library based upon the translation of bioactive IL-1 using rabbit reticulocyte lysates. Clones from this library were screened by hybridization selection of mRNA that translated bioactive IL-1 in the T lymphoma cell assay. A single large open reading frame that encoded a protein of 271 amino acids (Mr = 30,606 Da) was identified and termed IL-1α.

In a second cloning approach, March and co-workers purified a 17.5 kDa protein from LPS-activated human monocyte supernatants, and obtained a 13.5 kDa fragment from tryptic digests that yielded 26 amino acid residues, from which a 62 bp cDNA probe was constructed. This probe identified a 1,124 bp clone that defined a single large open reading frame coding for 269 amino acids (Mr = 30,749 Da), which showed only limited homology to the sequence of IL-1α. A 17.5 kDa (153 amino acid residues) carboxy-terminal segment of the alleged 269 amino acid precursor protein yielded biological activity in both the lymphoma cell and thymocyte IL-1 bioassays, so that this protein segment was termed IL-1 beta (IL-1β). Comparison of the two human cDNA sequences revealed only 26% amino acid homology. Comparison with the murine IL-1 sequence reported by Lomedico's group, revealed that human IL-1α and the murine IL-1 shared 62% amino acid homology, while human IL-1β had only 30% homology with murine IL-1. Accordingly, from these data it appeared that the human IL-1 cDNA identified could be homologous to the murine IL-1α.

Comparison of the three-reported human cDNAs revealed that the cDNA first reported by Dinarello's group was almost identical with the March group's IL1β cDNA, with only 7 nucleotide differences in the 3' non-translated region. Thus, either there were allelic differences or sequencing errors that could have accounted for these minor nucleotide differences. Northern blot analysis with cDNA probes encoding IL-1α and IL-1β of RNA from unstimulated and LPS-stimulated macrophages showed that LPS markedly augmented expression of both IL-1α and IL-1β mRNA as expected, and that IL-1β mRNA was ~10-fold in excess of IL-1α mRNA. From these data, it was not evident as to why these authors chose to designate one sequence IL-1α and the other IL-1β, however both recombinant proteins were detectable in the murine thymocyte IL-1 bioassay as well as the lymphoma cell assay, and both had endogenous pyrogen activity in the rabbit fever bioassay.

Accordingly, all these investigators felt that they had identified cDNAs encoding IL-1 activity, but it was left to conjecture whether they all interacted with T cells via the same putative receptor to account for the similar bioactivity. Moreover, the microheterogeneity noted in earlier experiments suggested that perhaps there might be a whole family of molecules with IL-1 activity.

Elucidation of the Structures of MHC Genes and their Products

The determination of the primary structures of the MHC genes originated in Jack Strominger's laboratory.[60] Surface molecules from lymphoblastoid cells were purified using immunoaffinity columns constructed from antisera reactive with β2 microglobulin (12 kDa), and then peptides from cyanogen bromide cleavage yielded fragments of the 44 kDa (Heavy Chain) component that could be sequenced, so that the carboxy-terminal 30 amino acids were determined in 1978. In 1980,

Strominger's group was then first to isolate a partial cDNA clone that encoded a portion of HLA-B7.[61] Subsequently, in 1981 Sherman Weissman's group synthesized a 12 nucleotide primer based on Strominger's 1978 amino acid sequence and used it to extend a 30 nucleotide DNA probe that identified a cDNA clone from a library that corresponded to known HLA-B7 amino acid sequences.[62] In 1981, Leroy Hood's group used the same human DNA probe from Weissman's lab to interrogate two mouse cDNA libraries constructed from two distinct murine lymphoma cell lines, and identified three cDNA clones that encoded three distinct MHC gene products based upon their predicted amino acid sequences.[63] A striking homology was found between the cDNA sequences of the mouse MHC genes with the constant region domains of the mouse immunoglobulin μ gene, but there was no evidence for DNA rearrangement. Concomitantly, Philippe Kourisky's group also identified a cDNA clone encoding a mouse H^2 antigen.[64] Subsequently, just a few months later, Hood's group reported the isolation of a mouse genomic DNA sequence that encoded eight exons, which correlated with the structural domains of the murine transplantation antigen.[65] To determine the extent of the genomic region encoding Class I MHC genes, Hood's group constructed a cosmid DNA library containing large inserts (32–46 kb) of Balb/c sperm DNA, and used cosmid clones to demonstrate at least 36 Class I MHC genes in the mouse genome, spanning 837 kb of DNA.[66]

Class II MHC molecules, also called *I* region-associated or Ia antigens, are encoded by the *I* region of the MHC, which is localized between the regions encoding Class I genes, as determined by classic genetic experiments using MLCs between recombinant inbred strains of mice (for review see Ref. 34). As detailed in Chapters 1 and 2,[7,67] Ia antigens on the surface of macrophages and B-cells were found to be responsible for T cell activation by alloantigens and also to be responsible for genetic restriction of both peptide antigen-specific T cell proliferation,[31] as well as antibody production by AFCs.[32] The two biochemically well characterized Ia antigens, from the *I*-regions designated I-A and I-E, were found to be heterodimers composed of a 33–35-kDa α-chain and a 28–31-kDa β-chain. In addition, an *I*-J sub-region, located between the I-A and I-E regions was reported to encode one or more soluble T-cell-derived antigen-specific 'factors' released by activated T cells that *suppressed* immune responses. Indeed, early on many thought these antigen-specific suppressor factors to be soluble, secreted T cell antigen receptors, like antibodies are secreted B cell antigen receptors.

To extend the analysis of the genomic structure of the MHC Class I genes to the Class II region, in 1982 Hood's group used human-specific α-chain and β-chain cDNAs to probe the cosmid mouse genomic library and identified 18 overlapping cosmid clones representing about 200 kb of DNA from the *I*-region. Most important, correlation of the molecular map with the genetic map of the *I*-region resulted in two of the five *I* sub-regions, I-J and I-B, relegated to less than 3.4 kb of DNA, indicating that the I-J sub-region could not be encoded in the MHC *I*-region. From this point on, the whole concept of "Suppressor T cells" that secreted I-J-encoded antigen-specific "Suppressor Factors" degenerated and rapidly disappeared as an active research area of immunology.

The molecular genetic approaches allowed insight for the first time into the molecular mechanisms of the extreme polymorphism of MHC Class I and Class II molecules. From the sequence information, it became clear that most of the polymorphism occurs in the first two external domains of the molecules, such that the third domain was much more highly conserved. Genetic engineering also opened the way to mutational immunogenetic experiments that promised to further understanding of just how MHC encode molecules restricted immune responses as well as how they led to "high & low responders." However, it was not until new structural biology approaches were applied to MHC encoded molecules that the nature of the "peptide-MHC complex" became understood for the 1st time. Pamela Bjorkman, working in the late 80s as a joint graduate student between two mentors, Jack Strominger and Donald Wiley, showed the way. The team grew hundreds of liters of EBV-transformed B lymphoblastoid cell lines derived from consanguineous individuals that only expressed one HLA-A allele and one HLA-B allele, and purified mg quantities of purified HLA molecules obtained after papain cleavage. These purified proteins were used to form crystals that could be used for X-Ray diffraction studies. The results, published in 1987 in two seminal articles,[68,69] revealed the structure of MHC Class I-encoded molecules showing how two parallel alpha helices from the first and second external domains formed a groove that could be occupied by a foreign oligopeptide, so that together the two molecules formed an antigenic peptide-MHC complex that could be recognized by one T cell antigen receptor (TCR) complex.

Subsequent studies revealed that endogenous "self" peptides are normally present in the alpha helical groove, so that TCRs must somehow scan the surface of cells and only become activated when there is a high affinity or avidity interaction between the TCR and the peptide-MHC, or when there is an unusually high density of peptide-MHC complexes that could activate a TCR with a lower affinity or avidity.

Antigen Processing

Given that Baruj Benacerraf found as early as 1963 that peptides could be antigenic, driving a Delayed Type Hypersensitvity response,[70] and as early as 1966 Stuart Schlossman found that only six amino acid residues were sufficient,[28] with the advances in cellular immunology over the 1970s, by the 1980s the stage was set to elucidate the mechanisms whereby APCs process large proteins into peptides that could be recognized ultimately by T cells as peptide-MHC complexes (pMHC). The first inkling that APCs actually process antigenic proteins to peptides was provided by Kirk Ziegler and Emil Unanue in 1981.[71] To approach events occurring in APCs within minutes after antigen ingestion, these investigators used an assay based upon binding of antigen-specific T cells to antigen-loaded APCs. Prior to that time, antigen activation was monitored by the T cell proliferative response, which occurred days later. Beginning in 1975, several investigators had studied the phenomenon of T cell-APC binding. Ziegler and Unanue quantified this interaction, so that one could approach detailed kinetic experiments, focusing on a much more abbreviated time scale.[72] The binding of immune T cells was monitored by the absorption of T cell mediated cytotoxicity using *Listeria monocytogenes*-exposed macrophages vs.

control antigen exposed macrophages. Using such an assay, these investigators could study the uptake, ingestion, and catabolism of *Listeria* as a function of time. Substantial uptake occurred within 5–10 minutes, while the ingestion occurred almost concomitantly, and catabolism of radiolabeled *Listeria* occurred with a $t^{1/2} \sim 2$ hours. In further studies, Ziegler and Unanue showed that the uptake and ingestion of *Listeria* by macrophages were not affected by two lysosomotropic compounds, ammonia and chloroquine, but macrophage catabolism of ^{125}I-labeled *Listeria* was reduced in a dose-dependent manner, as was antigen presentation to T cells as monitored by the macrophage-T cell binding assay.[73]

If antigenic foreign peptides resulted from APC processing of larger proteins, then one would anticipate that already processed peptides would bind to isolated purified MHC-encoded molecules. Again, Unanue's group provided the definitive data in a 1985 report.[74] As antigen, the 15 amino acid peptide from Hen Eggwhite Lysozyme (HEL),[46-61] which was fluorescently labeled with 7-fluoro-4-nirobenzo-2-oxa-1,3-diazole (NBD) was used. MHC Class II encoded molecules from 10^{11} B cell hybridoma cells that expressed I-A^k and I-A^d were purified via monoclonal antibody immunoaffinity chromatography. The association of the MHC molecules and the NBD-HEL[46-61] was them quantified via equilibrium dialysis. The binding was specific for I-A^k molecules, was saturable, and of a reasonable affinity ($K_d \sim 2$ µM). However, given this relatively low affinity, it became obvious that a high intracellular concentration of foreign peptide would have to be processed to "arm" an APC so that a reactive T cell could be stimulated.

In 1986, Thomas Braciale's group provided the first evidence that antigen processing and presentation differed between MHC Class I and MHC Class II molecules.[75] Building on Gunter Dennert's 1981 observation that cloned murine Lyt2$^+$(CD8)-negative IA-restricted T cells demonstrated both cytolytic as well as helper capacities,[76] and Ellis Reinherz's 1982 data that cloned human CD4+ T cells could be cytolytic,[77] Braciale's group examined requirements for antigen presentation to a panel of Class I and Class II-restricted, influenza-specific CTL clones by controlling the form of virus presented on the target cell surface. Both Class I-and Class II-region restricted CTL recognized target cells exposed to infectious virus, but only the Class II-restricted CTL clones efficiently lysed histocompatible target cells pulsed with inactivated virus preparations. Furthermore, isolated influenza hemagglutinin polypeptide could sensitize target cells for recognition by Class II-restricted CTL, but not Class I-restricted CTL. In addition, inhibition of nascent viral protein synthesis abrogated the capacity of target cells to present viral antigen relevant for Class I-restricted CTL recognition. Moreover, treatment of target cells with the lysosomotropic agent chloroquine abolished recognition of infected target cells by Class II-restricted CTL without diminishing Class I-restricted killing.

All these data established that, (1) T cell-mediated functions of cytotoxicity and help are not mutually exclusive T cell functions, predictable by MHC restriction, (2) that MHC-restriction is mediated by the T cell exclusive expression of two co-receptor molecules, CD4 and CD8, and (3) that processing and presentation of peptides via either MHC Class I or Class II occurs through distinct metabolic pathways.

Lymphotoxin (LT) and Tumor Necrosis Factor (TNF)

Soon after the 1965 reports of a mitogenic factor activity in the culture supernatants of mitogen/alloantigen-stimulated lymphocytes,[14,15] in 1968 Gale Granger and T.W. Williams reported that these same kinds of supernatants would lyse target L cells. Control supernatants prepared from unstimulated lymphocytes were ineffective, and the Lymphocyte Cytotoxic Factor (LCF) activity of the culture supernatants correlated with the appearance of blast cells.[78] This phenomenon was corroborated by Nancy Ruddle and Byron Waksman, also in 1968, who found that lymphocytes from tuberculin-sensitized rat lymph node cells released a soluble factor cytotoxic for rat fibroblasts when stimulated in vitro by purified protein derivative.[79] Ruddle and Waksman quantified the cytolytic activity by counting supernatant-treated fibroblasts remaining after 72 hours, while Granger and Williams utilized C^{14}-labeled amino acid uptake after 48 hours of culture. Subsequently, William Kolb and Granger reported the initial biochemical characteristics of human and mouse cytotoxic activities that they termed *Lymphotoxin* (LT): the activity was heat sensitive, pH stable, and trypsin, RNAase and DNAase-insensitive, with an approximate molecular size of ~85 kDa.[80]

Initially, it was assumed that the LT activity was released by lymphocytes, hence the name. However, in 1971 Peter Alexander reported that murine macrophage monolayers became cytotoxic for lymphoma cells when cultured with lipopolysaccharide (LPS), double-stranded (ds) RNA, or synthetic polyribonucleotides such as Poly-I:Poly-C. Moreover, the induced cytotoxic activity appeared in the culture supernatants as a soluble activity that required at least 12 hours of incubation.[81] These investigators conjectured that per- haps "*there is a receptor in the membrane of macrophages which is activated by both ds RNA and lipid A.*" (from LPS)

In this regard, it is important to mention that in 1893 William Coley first reported that bacteria as well as bacterial extracts could cause necrosis of tumors in humans.[82] Subsequently, over the first half of the 20th century, investigators had identified one of the effec- tive bacterial components as LPS.[83,84] Then in 1975, Lloyd Old's group reported that mice infected with the mycobacteria Bacillus Calmette Guerin (BCG),[85] which induced hyperplasia of the reticu- loendothelial system (RES), when injected 14–21 days with LPS, resulted in circulatory shock, and the appearance in the serum of an activity that they termed Tumor Necrosis Factor (TNF).[86] Serum taken from these animals within 2–4 hours after the LPS injection induced hemorrhagic necrosis of chemically induced tumors of test mice. Of note, the test tumors had to be quite large and the necrosis would peak 24 hours after the TNF serum injection. No TNF activity was detected if either BCG or LPS were given alone. Also, mixed bacterial vaccines and poly-I: poly-C could be substituted for LPS, while old tuberculin or *B. abortis* could not.

Because these investigators found that the same sera containing TNF activity were cytotoxic for *L* cells *in vitro*, they concluded that the effects observed *in vivo* of hemorrhagic necrosis were due to the TNF and not due to the hypotension caused via the LPS injections.

Although this report was seven years after the first reports of LT activity, which had become routinely assayed via L cells, these investigators did not mention the possibility that LT and TNF might be synonymous. However, they did monitor for interferon (IFN) activity of partially purified TNF preparations, and found no antiviral activity, thereby excluding it as responsible. Also, they suggested perhaps "*TNF mediates the selective* (i.e. tumor) *toxicity of* (LPS)-*activated macrophages*" described earlier by Alexander and Evans.[81] Subsequent biochemical analysis of TNF activity in mouse sera via ammonium sulfate precipitation, molecular gel filtration, and preparative polyacrylamide gel electrophoresis indicated that the active component is made up of at least four subunits with a molecular size of ~150 kDa.[87]

Even before these findings, the *acute phase response* had been described as a series of changes in circulating cells and serum proteins following infection with a variety of microbes (bacterial, viral, protozoan, and metazoans) as well as some tumors. These changes included fever, leukocytosis, and elevated concentrations of specific serum proteins such as fibrinogen, haptoglobin, and serum amyloid A protein. In addition, investigators interested in metabolism had noted hyperlipidemia in association with infections and cancer. In 1981, Masanobu Kawakami and Anthony Cerami reported that the hyperlipidemia that occurs in LPS-injected mice resulted from the release of a "humoral mediator factor" from peritoneal exudate cells (~60% macrophages) that functioned to decrease lipoprotein lipase activity in adipose tissues.[88] The molecular nature of this soluble factor was left unexplored, as was the mechanism of the decrease in membrane lipoprotein lipase activity.

Then, in 1984 Bharat Aggarwal and co-workers isolated and purified a molecule with LT activity from the supernatants of a human lymphoblastoid cell line (RPMI-1788).[89] Cells were cultured in serum-free media for 65 hours, and it is noteworthy that no mention was made that any stimuli were used to induce the LT production. Starting from a huge amount of conditioned media, approximately ~300 L, a protein with LT activity determined by a quantitative L-929 cell bioassay was purified 20,000-fold to apparent homogeneity, as determined by polyacrylamide gel electrophoresis under native and denaturing conditions and by gel permeation HPLC. The purified LT had a Mr of ~60,000 by gel permeation chromatography, and under denaturing conditions it migrated as a 20 kDa species, thereby indicating that the native LT activity might be attributable to a homotrimer. From the data reported, the starting 294 L contained only 250 µg LT protein, for an initial concentration of only 0.85 µg/L. Because the various biochemical separative processes resulted in a loss of ~90% of the starting LT activity, only 25 µg of purified homogeneous LT protein remained.

Despite the low yield of purified human LT protein, later in 1984 Aggarwal's team purified enough LT protein from RPMI 1788 cells that migrated on SDS polyacrylamide gels as two bands of Mr 25 kDa (~95% of material) and ~20 kDa (~5% of material).[90] Microsequencing of the 25 kDa material led to the synthesis of a cDNA probe that was then used by Patrick Gray's team to isolate a natural LT cDNA clone. Northern and Southern blot analysis provided evidence for a single mRNA transcript encoded by a single gene. Polyclonal antibodies prepared in rabbits against natural LT neutralized all of the cytolytic activity produced by recombinant LT (rLT). rLT purified via a MoAb immunoaffinity column migrated at Mr 18 kDa consistent with the predicted value of 18,600 based on the deduced amino acid sequence. The rLT was cytotoxic to L-cells $in vitro$ and of significance, caused significant necrosis of MethA sarcomas $in vivo$. The predicted amino acid sequence of rLT compared with the sequences of the other known cytokine sequences of interferon-γ (INF-γ), IL-2 and IL-3 revealed no significant homologies, so that this represented a new lymphokine molecule.

Bharat Aggarwal also identified a cytokine derived from adherent human peripheral blood mononuclear cells (PBMC) when activated by a combination of BCG and LPS, stimuli used originally to demonstrate TNF activity.[91] Because non-adherent PBMCs, primarily lymphocytes, did not produce this activity, and because anti-LT did not neutralize the cytolytic activity it appeared that a distinct molecule was responsible. A promyelocytic leukemia cell line (HL60) was found to produce the TNF cytolytic activity when treated with

4β-phorbol 12β-myristate 13α-acetate (PMA). Batches of 50–100 L of HL60 conditioned media were purified to apparent homogeneity, and tryptic peptides were sequenced, yielding a 42 bp cDNA that was used to probe an HL60-derived cDNA library.[92] From the deduced amino acid sequences derived from several cDNA clones identified, it appeared that a mature sequence of 17,356 (*Mr*) is derived from a precursor, and that a single gene encodes a single 18S mRNA transcript. Both rTNF and nTNF had cytolytic activity tested on *L*-929 cells *in vitro* and on MetA sarcomas *in vivo*. It was also noteworthy that 44 of the 157 TNF amino acid residues (28%) correspond to LT residues, thereby confirming the suspicion that the two cytotoxins are analogous, but not identical.

Concomitantly, in 1985 Bruce Beutler working in Anthony Cerami's group, purified cachectin to homogeneity from the conditioned media of an LPS-activated murine macrophage cell line (RAW 264.7).[93] Such conditioned media were found to suppress the activity of lipoprotein lipase (LPL) by the selective inhibition of LPL biosynthesis in the adipocyte cell line 3T3-L1. A quantitative 3T3-L1 cachectin bioassay was used to purify the active moiety from ~10L conditioned media, using preparative isoelectric focusing, Con-A Sepharose chromatography and non-denaturing PAGE. The resultant purified protein yielded a monomeric *Mr* of ~17 kDa. It is noteworthy that radioiodinated cachectin apparently interacted with specific, high affinity (K_d = 33 nM) hormone-like receptors present on many normal murine tissues, including adipocytes, muscle and liver membranes. Purified cachectin lacked IL-1 or IL-2 activity, but subsequent studies revealed by N-terminal amino acid sequencing of cachectin a *"striking homology with the N-terminal sequence of human TNF: all but 5 of the first 19 residues are in agreement."*[94] Accordingly, all these data indicated that TNF/cachectin mediated marked hormone-like metabolic activity on diverse normal tissues so that this molecule and its receptor were not confined to simply cytolysis of tumor cells.

In view of finding that murine cachectin/TNF bound to receptors present on several normal (non-transformed) murine tissues, and capable of evoking a biochemical response (LPL suppression in adipocytes), Beutler and Cerami suggested for the first time that *"cachectin/TNF, when elaborated in vivo, elicits specific (physio-logic) metabolic responses in various normal host tissues."* Thus, the effects of this newly discovered hormone-like molecule and its receptor could no longer be considered as confined solely to host defenses against tumor cells. As noted by Kawakami and Cerami in their first publication regarding cachectin, there was no loss of LPL activity in C3H/HeJ mice provoked by LPS, which were known to be resistant to LPS-induced shock, in contrast to C3H/HeN mice, which were susceptible.[88] Subsequently, Beutler, Milsark and Cerami pas-sively immunized mice with rabbit antibody reactive with murine cachectin/TNF and then challenged them with lethal amounts of LPS.[95] Maximal protection of the antisera was obtained if given before the injection of the LPS, and it was noteworthy that although protected from the lethal effects of LPS, the treated mice still became febrile and appeared ill and distressed. Thus, it was interpreted that cachectin/TNF was only one of the mediators released after LPS administration, leading to the conjecture that other mediators such as IL-1, IFN, and LT might also contribute to the pathologic picture of sepsis.

In 1986, to test directly the hypothesis that cachectin/TNF was responsible for the lethal effects of bacterial endotoxin (LPS), Beutler and Cerami collaborated with Kevin Tracey working in Thomas Shires' surgical group.[96] Thus, recombinant cachectin/TNF was expressed in yeast, purified to homogeneity and infused intrave-nously (IV) in rats. Animals receiving in excess of 600-µg/Kg-body weight became lethargic within minutes after infusion, followed by piloerection, bloody diarrhea, and tachypnea. In further experiments rats treated with cachectin underwent pathophysiological and histo-logical changes identical to those routinely found after the adminis-tration of bacterial endotoxin. Thus, inflammatory pneumonitis, mesenteric ischemia with infarction, and acute renal tubular necrosis seen after cachectin infusion were pathognomonic of septic shock observed after LPS administration. Moreover, LPS contamination of the purified cachectin was excluded as causative by the prophylactic administration of anti-cachectin MoAb, which prevented the syndrome.

In further 1986 experiments, Charles Dinarello, in collaboration with both the cachectin group, as well as the TNF group, found that purified homogeneous cachectin/TNF had endogenous pyrogen (EP) activity in the *in vivo* fever assay, and in addition induced the production of IL-1 both *in vitro* and *in vivo*.[97] Noteworthy, pure cachectin/TNF scored positive in the thymocyte proliferation assay, but only when IL-1 was neutralized with MoAb. Thus, these experiments reconciled many of the conflicting findings regarding EP activities, showing that several molecules could induce fever, and that putative adjuvant activities of cachectin/TNF might be indirect, ascribable to its capacity to induce IL-1 production by macrophages.

The Interferons (IFN)

Like the mitogenic factors described in lymphocyte conditioned media derived from mixed leukocyte cultures,[14,15] in 1965 Fred Wheelock found that similar conditioned media derived from PHA-stimulated human leukocytes contained an antiviral activity.[98] The characteristics of the activity were similar to the antiviral activities found in culture supernatants upon New Castle Disease virus infection, i.e. not sedimented by ultracentrifugation, indicating a soluble molecule(s), but differing by sensitivity to both acid and alkaline pH, and to mild heat (56°C). These physicochemical characteristics were used subsequently to identify this apparently unique antiviral activity thereafter, especially the acid sensitivity. Subsequently in 1969, Jon Green working with Sidney Cooperband and Sydney Kibrick showed that human peripheral blood mononuclear cells produce interferon (IFN) activity when immune donor cells are stimulated *in vitro* by non-viral antigens such as Purified Protein Derivative (PPD) and Tetanus Toxoid.[99] Thus, this IFN was designated "Immune IFN" or Type II IFN to distinguish it from virally-induced IFN, which came to be called Type I IFN.

Experiments designed to explore additional effects of IFN besides the antiviral activity, began to pick up pace in the 1970s. Thus, Ion Gresser and coworkers found in 1970 that IFN preparations had antiproliferative activity *in vitro* on cultured murine leukemia cells (L1210),[100] and then followed this observation by showing that IFN preparations also inhibited PHA- or allogeneic lymphocyte-stimulated murine lymphocyte proliferation *in vitro* in 1972.[101] Accordingly, this IFN anti-proliferative activity was not confined to malignant cells, as some investigators hoped, but seemed as though it was a generalized anti-cellular property. My own experiments on the IFN effect of suppressing erythropoietin-stimulated fetal liver cell proliferation confirmed and extended this interpretation to another normal cell type, as well as providing a plausible explanation of anemia observed during viral infections and chronic inflammatory syndromes.[102]

Subsequently, in 1973 Gresser's group using the absorptive capacity of cytotoxic alloantisera showed that IFN preparations enhanced the expression of surface antigens on murine L1210 leukemia cells.[103] In this report, it was not defined whether the cell surface antigen detected were histocompatibility molecules, but subsequent experiments by Gresser's group found enhanced expression of histocompatibility antigens on lymphoid cells of mice treated with IFN.[104] Subsequently, in 1977 Francois Vignaux and Gresser showed that Type I IFN promoted only the expression of Class-I MHC encoded antigens, but not Class-II MHC encoded antigens on murine lymphocytes.[105] Then, in 1980 Patricia Steeg with Joost Oppenheim showed quite unequivocally that Con-A murine splenocyte conditioned media promoted a dose-dependent increase in the percentage of MHC Class-II (Ia)+ phagocytic peritoneal exudate cells.[106]

Obviously, the IFN field suffered from the lack of homogeneous purified IFN molecules, and the molecular characteristics of Type-I and Type-II IFN remained unknown because analytical biochemical methods were not very precise. Although the antiviral IFN bioassays were quantitative, purification efforts had failed because of the scarcity of IFN molecules in active supernatants, compounded by the large amounts of contaminating serum proteins. A breakthrough occurred in 1980 when Michael Hunkapiller and Leroy Hood improved the sensitivity of automated amino acid analysis ~10,000-fold so that only μg rather than mg quantities of purified proteins could be sequenced.[107] To demonstrate the power of this new technique, human fibroblast (Type-I) IFN produced in serum-free media was purified using a combination of Blue Sepharose and preparative SDS-polyacrylamide gel electrophoresis. Thus, 10–15 L of IFN-containing media yielded 5–10 µg of homogeneous protein, enough to determine the sequence of the first 13 amino-terminal amino acids.[108] Concomitantly in 1980, Kathryn Zoon working with Christian Anfinsen's group collaborated with Hunkapillar and Hood, and found that IFN purified from B-lymphoblastoid cells stimulated with Newcastle disease virus yielded an 18.5 kDa protein that differed from the human fibroblast IFN in the initial N-terminal amino acid sequence.[109]

With the advent of cDNA cloning, an alternative approach to the determination of the primary structures of biologically important proteins became available, and Charles Weissmann's group in collaboration with Kari Cantell's laboratory reported in 1980 that IFN derived from 100 billion Sendai virus-induced peripheral blood leukocytes ultimately resulted in a 910 bp cDNA that selected leukocyte mRNA that produced IFN antiviral activity when injected into Xenopus oocytes.[110] Determination of the nucleotide sequence of this cDNA predicted an IFN polypeptide of 166 amino acids (MW = 19,390 Da), and a comparison of 35 predicted amino-terminal amino acids revealed nine differences from the lymphoblastoid-derived IFN reported by Zoon et al.,[109] thereby suggesting that two separate genes encoded these IFNs.[111] Thus, even though "leukocytes" or white blood cells were used in both instances, two ostensibly different genes seemed responsible, so that it became apparent that a family of genes could be responsible for distinct gene products, all of which had antiviral activity. Concomitantly in 1980, Tadatsugu Taniguchi, used similar approaches to identify and clone an IFN cDNA derived from human fibroblasts. For these experiments, 2 billion human diploid fibroblasts were stimulated to produce IFN activity with poly(I)-poly(C)+ cycloheximide. A cDNA was found to encode IFN activity by hybridization selection of mRNA that produced IFN activity when translated by Xenopus oocytes, and also when translated via rabbit reticulocyte lysates.[112,113] It is noteworthy that the predicted amino acid sequences of the leukocyte, lymphoblastoid and fibroblast IFNs all differed from one another.

Weissmann's group then reported at least eight distinct genes encoding IFN activity, isolated from a genomic DNA of single individual, thereby indicating that there are multiple leukocyte IFN genes.[114] Simultaneously in 1980, Geoffrey Allen and Karl Fantes reported that leukocyte IFN consists of a family of proteins with at least five different, but homologous, primary structures.[115] This report was followed in 1981 by a confirmation from David Goeddel working in Patrick Gray's group.[116] Thus, all these data indicated that of the two major classes of human type I IFNs, leukocyte IFN (IFN-α) activities were due to the products of multiple genes, whereas fibroblast IFN (IFN-β) could be attributed to only one gene.

By this time considerably less structural data had accumulated on "immune IFN" or IFNγ. IFNγ was characterized as produced in lymphocyte cultures exposed to various mitogenic stimuli rather than viruses or polyribonucleotides, i.e., the same source of all the other lymphokine or cytokine activities found to date. Also, IFNγ activity differed from IFNα and IFNβ activities by its susceptibility to an acid pH, and by not cross-reacting with antisera reactive with either IFNα or IFNβ. Accordingly, in 1982 Patrick Gray's group produced IFNγ activity from human peripheral blood lymphocytes stimulated by staphylococcal enterotoxin B, and isolated a cDNA encoding IFNγ activity by similar procedures used for the other IFNs.[117] This cDNA encoded IFN activity when expressed either in *E. coli* or monkey kidney cells that was not neutralized by anti-IFNα or anti-IFN-β, but was neutralized by anti-IFNγ. Furthermore, consistent with these findings the rIFNγ was neutralized by treatment with acid pH, while the other two IFNs were not. The cDNA sequence predicted an amino acid sequence that was not homologous with either IFNα or IFNβ, except at one 4-amino acid site. The 146 amino acid polypeptide estimated to contain the mature protein had a calculated molecular weight of 17,110, smaller than the molecular weights of either of the other IFNs. Thus, IFNγ was found to be chemically as well as biologically distinct from IFNα and IFNβ.[118] Similar findings were also reported by Walter Fiers and co-workers, thereby confirming these IFNγ characteristics.[119]

Accordingly, over the course of thirty years, between 1960 and 1990, the roles of antigen presenting cells were finally clearly defined at the molecular level. In addition to protein antigen ingestion, digestion, processing and presentation of short peptides bound firmly by MHC gene products, the histocompatibility molecules, macrophages produce immunoactive cytokines, including interleukins, cytotoxins and interferons that markedly augment the functions of all the participating cells, including the macrophages/antigen-presenting cells, T cells and B cells. Over the ensuing decades beginning in the 1990s, the cell surface receptors of the cytokines, their signaling pathways and the genes activated by the cytokines were exhaustively defined at the molecular level. However, the keys to all these molecular developments were the identification and characterization of the initiator molecules, the cytokines and the MHC encoded molecules. Also during these years, notable was the characterization of dendritic cells as "professional APCs" after their cultivation *in vitro* using cytokines in the 1990s. However, it is significant that their professional APC functions were not attributable to the discovery of new APC molecules, but rather to the enhanced expression of those molecules already discovered.

References

1. Metchnikoff E. (1905). *Immunity in Infective Diseases.* Cambridge, UK: Cambridge University Press, 576 pp.
2. Behring EAS and Kitasato S. (1890). Ueber das zustandekommen der diphtherie-immunaitat und der tetanus-immunitat bei thieren. *DMW* 16:113–114.
3. Fagraeus A. (1948). The plasma cellular reaction and its relation to the formation of antibodies *in vitro. J Immunol* 58:1–13.
4. Jerne NK. (1955). The natural selection theory of antibody formation. *Proc Natl Acad Sci USA* 41:849–857.
5. Burnet FM. (1957). A modification of Jerne's theory of antibody production using the concept of clonal selection. *Aust J Sci* 20: 67–77.
6. Jerne NK and Nordin AA. (1963). Antibody formation in agar by single antibody-producing cells. *Science* 140:405.
7. Smith K. (2012). Toward a molecular understanding of adaptive immunity: A chronology, Part I. *Front Immun* 3:369.
8. Mishell R and Dutton R. (1967). Immunization of dissociated spleen cell cultures from normal mice. *J Exp Med* 126:423–442.

9. Mosier D. (1967). A requirement for two cell types for antibody formation *in vitro. Science* **158**:1573–1575.

10. Ehrenreich B and Cohn Z. (1967). The uptake and digestion of iodinated human serum albumin by macrophages *in vitro. J Exp Med* **126**:941–962.

11. Unanue E and Askonas BA. (1968). Persistence of immunogenicity of antigen after uptake by macrophages. *J Exp Med* 127.

12. Unanue E, Cerottini J, and Bedford M. (1969). Persistence of antigen on the surface of macrophages. *Nature* **222**:1193–1195.

13. Unanue E and Cerottini J. (1970). The immunogenecity of antigen bound to the plasma membrane of macrophages. *J Exp Med* **131**:711–725.

14. Kasakura S and Lowenstein L. (1965). A factor stimulating DNA synthesis derived from the medium of leukocyte cultures. *Nature* **208**:794–795.

15. Gordon J and MacLean LD. (1965). A lymphocyte-stimulating factor produced *in vitro. Nature* **208**:795–796.

16. Bach F, Alter B, Solliday S, *et al.* (1970). Lymphocyte reactivity *in vitro* II. Soluble reconstituting factor permitting response of purified lymphocytes. *Cell Immunol* **1**:219–227.

17. Hoffman M and Dutton R. (1971). Immune response restoration with macrophage culture supernatants. *Science* **172**:1047–1048.

18. Oppenheim J, Leventhal B, and Hersh E. (1968). The transformation of column-purified lymphocytes with nonspecific and specific antigenic stimuli. *J Immunol* **101**:262–270.

19. Gery I, Gershon RK, and Waksman B. (1972). Potentiation of the T-lymphocyte response to mitogens I. The responding cell. *J Exp Med* **136**:128–142.

20. Gery I and Waksman BH. (1972). Potentiation of the T-lymphocyte response to mitogens: The cellular source of potentiating mediators. *J Exp Med* **136**:143–155.

21. Chess L, Schmuckler M, Smith K, and Mardiney M. (1972). The effect of synthetic polyribonucleotides on immunologically induced tritiated thymidine incorporation. *Transplantation* **14**:748–756.

22. Schmidtke J and Johnson A. (1971). Regulation of the immune system by synthetic polynucleotides. I. Characteristics of adjuvant action on antibody synthesis. *J Immunol* **106**:1191–1200.

23. Cornell C, Smith K, Cornwell G, *et al.* (1976). Systemic effects of intravenous polyriboinosinic-polyribocytidylic acid in man. *J Natl Cancer Inst* **57**:1211–1216.

24. Bennett IJ and Beeson P. (1953). Studies on the pathogenesis of fever II. Characterization of fever producing substances from polymorphonuclear leukocytes and from the fluid of sterile exudates. *J Exp Med* **98**:493–508.

25. Bodel P and Atkins E. (1967). Release of endogenous pyrogen by human monocytes. *N Eng J Med* **276**:1002–1008.

26. Dinarello C, Goldin N, and Wolff S. (1974). Demonstration and characterization of two distinct human leukocyte pyrogens. *J Exp Med* **139**:1369–1381.

27. Kantor FS, Ojeda A, and Benacerraf B. (1963). Studies on artificial antigens I. Antigenicity of DNP-polylysine and DNP copolymer of lysine and glutamic acid in guinea pigs. *J Exp Med* **117**:55–64.

28. Schlossman S, Ben-Efraim S, Yaron A, and Sober H. (1966). Immunochemical studies on the antigenic determinants required to elicit delayed and immediate hypersensitivity reactions. *J Exp Med* **123**:1083–1095.

29. Green I, Paul W and Benacerraf B. (1966). The behavior of hapten-poly-L-lysine conjugates as complete antigens in genetic responder and as haptens in non-responder guinea pigs. *J Exp Med* **123**:859–879.

30. McDevitt HO and Tyan ML. (1968). Genetic control of the antibody response in inbred mice: Transfer of response by spleen cells and linkage to the major histocompatability (H2) locus. *J Exp Med* **128**:1–11.

31. Rosenthal A and Shevach E. (1973). Function of macrophages in antigen recognition by guinea pig T lymphocytes. I. Requirement for histocompatible macrophages and lymphocytes. *J Exp Med* **138**:1194–1212.

32. Katz D, Hamaoka T, and Benacerraf B. (1973). Cell interactions between histoincompatible T and B lymphocytes II. Failure of physiologic cooperative interactions between T and B lymphocytes from allogeneic donor strains in humoral response to hapten-protein conjugates. *J Exp Med* **137**:1405–1418.

33. Zinkernagel R and Doherty P. (1974). Restriction of *in vitro* T cell-mediated cytotoxicity in lymphocytic choriomeningitis within a syngeneic or semiallogeneic system. *Nature* **248**:701–702.

34. Benacerraf B. (1978). A hypothesis to relate the specificity of T-lymphocytes and the activity of I region-specific Ir genes in macrophages and B lymphocytes. *J Immunol* **120**:1809–1812.

35. Diamanstein T, Handschumacher R, Oppenheim J, *et al.* 1979. Letter to the editor: Nonspecific "lymphocyte activating" factors produced by macrophages. *J Immunol* **122**:2633–2635.

36. Unanue E, Kiely J, and Calderon J. (1976). The modulation of lymphocyte functions by molecules secreted by macrophages. *J Exp Med* **144**:155–166.

37. Dinarello C, Renfer L, and Wolff S. (1977). The production of antibody against human leukocytic pyrogen. *J Clin Invest* **60**:465–472.

38. Meltzer M and Oppenheim J. (1977). Bidirectional amplification of macrophage-lymphocyte interactions: Enhanced lymphocyte activation factor production by activated adherent mouse peritoneal cells. *J Immunol* **118**:77–82.

39. Koren H, Handwerger B, and Wunderlich J. (1975). Identification of macrophage-like characteristics in a cultured murine tumor line. *J Immunol* **114**:894–897.

40. Lachman L, Hacker M, Blyden G, and Handschumacher R. (1977). Preparation of lymphocyte-activating factor from continuous murine macrophage cell lines. *Cell Immunol* **34**:416–419.

41. Mizel S, Oppenheim J, and Rosenstreich D. (1978). Characterization of lymphocyte-activating factor (LAF) produced by the macrophage cell line, P388D1. I. Enhancement of LAF production by activated T lymphocytes. *J Immunol* **120**:1497–1503.

42. Mizel S, Oppenheim J, and Rosenstreich D. (1978). Characterization of lymphocyte-activating factor (LAF) produced by a macrophage cell line, P388D1. II. Biochemical characterization of LAF induced by activated T cells and LPS. *J Immunol* **120**:1504–1508.

43. Waksman B. (1979). Nonantigenic specific monokines and lymphokines influencing T and B cell functions. In *Second International Lymphokine Workshop. A* deWeck, F Kristensen and M. Landy editor. Ermatingen, Switzerland: Academic Press, p. 417.

44. Rosenwasser L, Dinarello C, and Rosenthal A. (1979). Adherent cell function in murine T-lymphocyte antigen recognition IV. Enhancement of murine T-cell antigen recognition by human leukocytic pyrogen. *J Exp Med* **150**:709–714.

45. Gillis S and Smith KA. (1977). Long term culture of tumour-specific cytotoxic T cells. *Nature* **268**:154–156.

46. Baker PE, Gillis S, and Smith KA. (1979). Monoclonal cytolytic T-cell lines. *J Exp Med* **149**:273–278.

47. Smith KA. (1980). T-cell growth factor. *Immunol Rev* **51**:337–357.

48. Oppenheim J, Nortoff H, Greenhill A, *et al*. (1980). Properties of human monocyte derived lymphocyte activating factor (LAF) and lymphocyte derived mitogenic factor (LMF). In: *Biochemical Characterization of*

Lymphokines: Proceedings of the Second International Lymphokine Workshop. A de Weck, F Kristensen and M Landy, editors. New York: Academic Press, Inc. 399–404.

49. Smith K, Gilbride K, and Favata M. (1980). Lymphocyte activating factor promotes T cell growth factor production by cloned murine lymphoma cells. *Nature* **287**:853–855.

50. Larsson E, Iscove N, and Coutinho A. (1980). Two distinct factors are required for T cell growth. *Nature* **283**:664–666.

51. Smith KA, Lachman LB, Oppenheim JJ, and Favata MF. (1980). The functional relationship of the interleukins. *J Exp Med* **151**: 1551–1556.

52. Letter (1979). Revised nomenclature for antigen-nonspecific T cell proliferation and helper factors. *J Immunol* **123**:2928–2929.

53. Mizel S and Mizel D. (1981). Purification to apparent homogeneity of murine interleukin-1. *J Immunol* **126**:834–837.

54. Mizel S, Dukovich M, and Rothstein J. (1983). Preparation of goat antibodies against interleukin-1: Use of an immunoadsorbant to purify interleukin-1. *J Immunol* **131**:1834–1837.

55. Lomedico P, Gubler U, Hellman C, *et al.* (1984). Cloning and expression of murine interleukin-1 cDNA in Escherichia coli. *Nature* **312**:458–462.

56. Kaye J, Gillis S, Mizel S, *et al.* (1984). Growth of a cloned helper T cell line induced by a monoclonal antibody specific for the antigen receptor: Interleukin-1 is required for the expression of receptors for interleukin-2. *J Immunol* **133**:1339–1345.

57. Auron P, Webb A, Rosenwasser L, *et al.* (1984). Nucleotide sequence of human monocyte interleukin-1 precursor cDNA. *Proc Natl Acad Sci USA* **81**:7907–7911.

58. March C, Mosley B, Larson A, *et al.* (1985). Cloning, sequence and expression of two distinct human interleukin-1 complementary DNAs. *Nature* **315**:641–647.

59. Conlon P. (1983). A rapid biologic assay for the detection of interleukin-1. *J Immunol* **131**:1280–1282.

60. Robb R, Terhorst C, and Strominger J. (1978). Sequence of the COOH-terminal hydrophilic region of histocompatibility antigens HLA-A2 and HLA-B7. *J Biol Chem* **253**:5319–5324.

61. Ploegh H, Orr H, and Strominger J. (1980). Molecular cloning of a human histocompatibility antigen cDNA fragment. *Proc Natl Acad Sci USA* **77**:6081–6085.

62. Sood A, Periera D, and Weissman S. (1981). Isolation and partial nucleotide sequence of a cDNA clone for human histocompatibility antigen HLA-B by use of an oligonucleotide primer. *Proc Natl Acad Sci USA* **78**:616–620.

63. Steinmetz M, Frelinger J, Hunkapiller T, *et al.* (1981). Three cDNA clones encoding mouse transplantation antigens: Homology to immunoglobulin genes. *Cell* **24**:125–134.

64. Kvist S, Bregegere F, Rask L, *et al.* (1981). cDNA clone encoding for part of a mouse H-2d major histocmpatibility antigen. *Proc Natl Acad Sci USA* **78**:2772–2776.

65. Moore K, Sher B, Sun Y, *et al.* (1982). DNA sequences of a gene encoding a Balb/c mouse Ld transplantation antigen. *Science* **215**:679–682.

66. Steinmetz M, Winoto A, Minard K, and Hood L. (1982). Clusters of genes encoding mouse transplantation antigens. *Cell* **28**:489–498.

67. Smith K. (2012). Toward a molecular understanding of adaptive immunity: A chronology, Part II. *Front Immunol* **3**:364.

68. Bjorkman PJ, Saper MA, Samaoui B, *et al.* (1987). Structure of the human class I histocompatability antigen, HLA-A2. *Nature* **329**:506–511.

69. Bjorkman P, Saper M, Samaraoui B, *et al.* (1987). The foreign antigen binding site and T cell recognition regions of class I histocompatability antigens. *Nature* **329**:512–518.

70. Levine B, Ojeda M, and Benacerraf B. (1963). Studies on artificial antigens III. The genetic control of the immune response to hapten poly-L-lysine conjugates in guinea pigs. *J Exp Med* **118**:953–957.

71. Ziegler K and Unanue E. (1981). Identification of a macrophage antigen-processing event required for I-region restricted antigen presentation to T lymphocytes. *J Immunol* **127**:1869–1875.

72. Ziegler K and Unanue E. (1979). The specific binding of Listeria monocytogenes-immuneT lymphocytes to macrophages. I. Quantitation and role of H-2 gene products. *J Exp Med* **150**:1143–1149.

73. Ziegler H and Unanue E. (1982). Decrease in macrophage antigen catabolism caused by ammonia and chloroquine is associated with inhibition of antigen presentation to T cells. *Proc Natl Acad Sci USA* **79**:175–178.

74. Babbitt B, Allen P, Matsueda G, *et al.* (1985). Binding of immunogenic peptides to Ia histocompatibility molecules. *Nature* **317**: 59–361.

75. Morrison L, Lukacher A, Braciale V, *et al.* (1986). Differences in antigen presentation to mHC Class I- and Class II-restricted influenza virus-specific cytolytic T lymphocyte clones. *J Exp Med* **163**:903–921.

76. Dennert G, Weiss S, and Warner J. (1981). T cells may express multiple activities: Specific allohelp, cytolysis, and delayed-type hypersensitivity are expressed by a cloned T cell line. *Proc Natl Acad Sci USA* **78**:4540–4543.

77. Meuer S, Schlossman S, and Reinherz E. (1982). Clonal analysis of human cytolytic T lymphocytes: T4+ and T8+ effector T cells recognize products of different major histocompatibility regions. *Proc Natl Acad Sci USA* **79**:4395–4399.

78. Granger G and Williams T. (1968). lymphocyte cytotoxicity *in vitro*: Activation and release of a cytotoxic factor. *Nature* **218**:1253–1254.

79. Ruddle N and Waksman B. (1968). Cytotoxicity mediated by soluble antigen and lymphocytes in delayed hypersensitivity. III. Analysis of mechanism. *J Exp Med* **128**:1267–1279.

80. Kolb W and Granger G. (1968). Lymphocyte *in vitro* cytotoxicity: Characterization of human lymphotoxin. *Proc Natl Acad Sci USA* **61**:1250–1255.

81. Alexander P and Evans R (1971). Endotoxin and double stranded RNA render macrophages cytotoxic. *Nature New Biol* **232**:76–78.

82. Coley W. (1893). The treatment of malignant tumors by repeated inoculations of erysipalas: With a report of ten original cases. *Am J Med Sci* **10**:487–511.

83. Gratia A and Linz R. (1931). Le phenomene de Swartzman dans le sarcome du cobaye. *C.R. Seances Soc Biol Ses Fil* **108**:427–428.

84. Shear M. (1944). Chemical treatment of tumors. IX. Reactions of mice with primary subcutaneous tumors to injection of a hemorrhage-producing bacterial polysaccharide. *J Natl Cancer Inst* **4**:461–476.

85. Calmette A, Guerin C, Weill-Halle B, *et al.* (1924). Essais d'immunisation contre l'infection tuberculeuse. *Bulliten de l'Academie de Medicine* **91**:787–796.

86. Carswell E, Old L, Kassel R, *et al.* (1975). An endotoxin-induced serum factor that causes necrosis of tumors. *Proc Natl Acad Sci USA* **72**:3666–3670.

87. Green S, Dobrjansky A, Carswell E, *et al.* (1976). Partial purification of a serum factor that causes necrosis of tumors. *Proc Natl Acad Sci USA* **73**:381–385.

88. Kawakami M and Cerami A. (1981). Studies of endotoxin-induced decrease in lipoprotein lipase activity. *J Exp Med* **154**:631–639.

89. Aggarwal B, Moffat B, and Harkins R. (1984). Human lymphotoxin: Production by a lymphoblastoid cell line, purification, and initial characterization. *J Biol Chem* **259**:686–691.

90. Gray P, Aggarwal B, Benton C, *et al*. (1984). Cloning and expression of a cDNA for human lymphotoxin, a lymphokine with tumour necrosis activity. *Nature* **312**:721–724.

91. Aggarwal B, Kohr W, Hass P, *et al*. (1985). Human tumor necrosis factor. *J Biol Chem* **260**:2345–2354.

92. Pennica D, Nedwin GE, Hayflick JS, *et al*. (1984). Human tumour necrosis factor: Precursor structure, expression and homology to lymphotoxin. *Nature* **312**:724–729.

93. Beutler B, Mahoney J, Le TN, *et al*. (1985). Purification of cachectin, a lipoprotein lipase-suppressing hormone secreted by endotoxin-induced RAW 264.7 cells. *J Exp Med* **161**: 984–995.

94. Beutler B, Greenwald D, Hulumes J, *et al*. (1985). Identity of tumour necrosis factor and the macrophage-secreted factor cachectin. *Nature* **316**:352–354.

95. Beutler B, Milsark I, and Cerami A. (1985). Passive immunization against cachectin/tumor necrosis factor protects mice from lethal effect of endotoxin. *Science* **229**:869–871.

96. Tracey K, Beutler B, Lowry S, *et al*. (1986). Shock and tissue injury induced by recombinant human cachectin. *Science* **234**:470–474.

97. Dinarello C, Cannon J, Wolff S, *et al*. (1986). Tumor necrosis factor (cachectin) is an endogenous pyrogen and induces production of interleukin 1. *J Exp Med* **163**: 1433–1450.

98. Wheelock E. (1965). Interferon-like virus inhibitor induced in human leukocytes by phytohemagglutinin. *Science* **149**:310–311.

99. Green J, Cooperband S, and Kibrick S. (1969). Immune specific induction of interferon production in cultures of human blood lymphocytes. *Science* **164**:1415–1417.

100. Gresser I, Brouty-Boye D, Thomas M-T, and Maciera-Coelho A. (1970). Interferon and cell division, I. Inhibition of the multiplication of mouse leukemia L1210 cells *in vitro* by interferon preparations. *Proc Natl Acad Sci USA* **66**:1052–1058.

101. Lindahl-Magnusson P, Leary P, and Gresser I. (1972). Interferon inhibits DNA synthesis in mouse lymphocyte suspensions induced by phytohemagglutinin or by allogeneic cells. *Nature New Biol* **237**: 120–121.

102. Smith K, Fredrickson T, Mobraaten L, and DeMaeyer E. (1977). The interaction of erythropoietin with fetal liver cells. II. Inhibition of the erythropoietin effect by interferon. *Exp Hemat* **5**:333–340.

103. Lindhahl P, Leary P, and Gresser I. (1973). Enhancement by interferon of the expression of surface antigens on murine leulemia L1210 cells. *Proc Natl Acad Sci USA* **70**:2785–2788.

104. Lindahl P, Gresser I, Leary P, and Tovey M. (1976). Enhanced expression of histocompatibility antigens of lymphoid cells in mice treated with interferon. *J Infect Dis* **133** Suppl:A66–68.

105. Vignaux F and Gresser I. (1977). Differential effects of interferon on the expression of H-2K, H-2D, and Ia antigens on mouse lymphocytes. *J Immunol* **118**:721–723.

106. Steeg P, Moore R, and Oppenheim J. (1980). Regulation of murine macrophage Ia-antigen expression by products of activated spleen cells. *J Exp Med* **152**:1734–1744.

107. Hunkapiller M and Hood L. (1980). New protein sequenator with increased sensitvity. *Science* **207**:523–525.

108. Knight E, Hunkapiller M, Korant B, *et al.* (1980). Human fibroblast interferon: Amino acid analysis and amino terminal amino acid sequence. *Science* **207**:525–526.

109. Zoon K, Smith M, Bridgen P, *et al.* (1980). Amino terminal sequence of the major component of human lymphoblastoid interferon. *Science* **207**:527–528.

110. Nagata S, Taira H, Hall A, *et al.* (1980). Synthesis in *E. coli* of a polypeptide with human leukocyte interferon activity. *Nature* **284**:316–320.

111. Mantei N, Schwartzstein M, Streuli M, *et al.* (1980). The nucleotide sequence of a cloned human leukocyte interferon cDNA. *Gene* **10**:1–10.

112. Taniguchi T, Ohno S, Fuji-Kuriyama Y, and Muramatsu M. (1980). The nucleotide sequence of human fibroblast interferon cDNA. *Gene* **10**:11–15.

113. Taniguchi T, Fuji-Kuriyama Y, and Muramatsu M. (1980). Molecular cloning of human interferon cDNA. *Proc Natl Acad Sci USA* **77**:4003–4006.

114. Nagata S, Mantei N, and Weissmann C. (1980). The structure of one of the eight or more distinct chromosomal genes for human interferon-a. *Nature* **284**:401–408.

115. Allen G and Fantes K. (1980). A family of structural genes for human lymphoblastoid (leukocyte-type) interferon. *Nature* **284**:408–411.

116. Goeddel D, Leung D, Dull T, *et al.* (1981). The structure of eight distinct cloned human leukocyte interferon cDNAs. *Nature* **290**:20–26.

117. Gray P, Leung D, Pennica D, *et al.* (1982). Expression of human immune interferon cDNA in E. coli and monkey cells. *Nature* **295**:503–508.

118. Gray P and Goeddel D. (1982). Structure of the human immune interferon gene. *Nature* **298**:859–863.
119. Devos R, Cherroutre H, Taya Y, *et al.* (1982). Molecular cloning of human immune interferon cDNA and its expression in eukaryotic cells. *Nucleic Acids Res* **10**:2487–2501.

7 Additional T Cell Signals: Co-stimulatory and Co-inhibitory

The "Second" Signal Required for T Cell Activation

The advances in APC biology in the 1970s and 1980s assigned the APC role in T cell activation to two functions, (1) presentation of foreign antigenic peptides bound to surface histocompatibility molecules, a requirement for TCR antigen recognition, and (2) the production of co-stimulatory immunoactive cytokines such as IL-1, IL-6 and TNF, found to markedly augment IL-2 production and consequently, subsequent T cell proliferation. However, there still remained a third APC contribution to T cell activation. In 1980, John Hansen produced a monoclonal antibody (MoAb) that recognized a determinant selectively expressed by the majority of T cells, but not by B cells or macrophages.[1] This MoAb, designated 9.3, immunoprecipitated a 44 kDa molecule from T cell surfaces. Hansen went on to show that the 9.3+ subset of T cells, ~50–80% of peripheral T cells, contributed "helper activity" to immunoglobulin production by pokeweed mitogen activated lymphocytes.[2] Jeffrey Ledbetter and co-workers followed in 1985 showing that MoAb 9.3 was not directly mitogenic for T cells, but when used as a co-stimulant for macrophage-depleted T cells, these MoAbs augmented anti-CD3-stimulated T cell proliferation.[3] Thus, these findings required a reductionist approach fashioning a model system that lacked APCs.

In 1987, Alejandro Aruffo and Brian Seed used the 9.3 MoAb to clone a cDNA encoding the 44 kDa molecule, which by then was designated CD28.[4] From the predicted primary amino acid sequence, it could be surmised that the CD28 molecule was a member of the

Ig superfamily, and that it was expressed on the cell surface as a homodimer. Then in 1989, Craig Thompson working with Ledbetter, Howard Young and Carl June, among others, showed that MoAb 9.3 augmented the production of IL-2 by as much as 5–50-fold, as well as TNF-α, granulocyte-macrophage colony stimulating factor (GM-CSF), lymphotoxin (LT), and interferon-γ (IFNγ) from anti-CD3-stimulated human T cells.[5]

The molecular mechanisms responsible for this CD28 effect became the next obvious subject for experimentation. Accordingly, in 1989 the June, Ledbetter, and Thompson group showed that the CD28 pathway stabilized the mRNA encoding some of these same lymphokines, i.e. IL-2, IFNγ, TNFα, and GM-CSF, but not the mRNA of other genes activated by anti-CD3 T cell activation.[6] Subsequently also in 1989, Arthur Weiss's group found that CD28 triggering also induced the formation of a protein complex that bound to a distinct site on the IL-2 gene that increased IL-2 enhancer activity ~ five-fold, so that it appeared that two mechanisms, one transcriptional and one post-transcriptional, were activated by the CD28 pathway, all serving to augment cytokine gene expression.[7]

Four years later, in 1993 Howard Young's group then elucidated that the CD28 Response Element (CD28RE) in the IL-2 gene was a Rel-specific RE, and that both RelA (p65) and c-Rel bind to it.[8] Ellen Rothenberg and her group then used a combination of techniques in the mid-'90s to show that IL-2 gene transcription is regulated by a nonhierarchical, cooperative enhancesome formed by three families of transcription factors, AP-1, NF-AT and Rel that drives IL-2 gene expression in an all-or-none (quantal or digital) fashion.[9,10] The TCR/CD3 complex activates the p65 subunit of the Rel family, Rel-A, which is present in an inactive form in the cytoplasm of resting T cells. Hsiou-Chi Liou's group then showed in 1999 that the genetic deletion of c-Rel markedly impaired both IL-2 and IL-2R expression upon anti-CD3 T cell activation, followed by ablation of T cell proliferation and cytolytic activity, which could be circumvented by exogenous IL-2.[11] Thus, IL-2 gene transcription is initiated by the TCR, via the enhancesome formed initially with RelA, AP-1 and NF-AT. However, for sustained and productive IL-2 gene transcription, the c-Rel subunit of the Rel family must be activated via the co-stimulatory molecule CD28 and the CD28RE. In this regard, it is noteworthy that removal or prevention of any one of these transcription factors, e.g. pharmacologically, by immunosuppressive drugs such as glucocorticoids, cyclosporin-A, or FK506, disrupts the enhancesome and aborts IL-2 gene transcription.

Accordingly, *four signals* are required for productive and sustained T cell activation: (1) pMHC-TCR/CD3, (2) co-stimulatory cytokines (IL-1, IL-6, TNF), (3) co-stimulatory surface molecules, CD28, and (4) IL-2/IL-2R. It follows that abrogation of any one of these signals would markedly attenuate the T cell proliferation and the T cell immune response.

B7 Molecules, the CD28 Ligands on APCs

In 1987, Lee Nadler's group including Gordon Freeman, immunized mice with anti-Ig activated splenocytes, and then differentially screened for antibody reactivity against activated vs. non-activated splenocytes. A MoAb, termed B7 was found reactive with a minor fraction of non-activated splenocytes, ~34 ± 10%, but ~75% of splenic-derived B cells activated for 3-days by anti-Ig.[12] The surface molecule identified by the B7 MoAb was ~60 kDa by SDS-PAGE. This group subsequently went on to identify and isolate a cDNA clone encoding the B7-reactive antigen in 1989, and the predicted primary amino acid sequence indicated a type-I membrane protein of 262 amino acids.[13] The extracellular region was homologous to the Ig gene superfamily, with two contiguous Ig-like domains. While the predicted size was only 30 kDa, there were eight potential N-linked glycosylation sites.

Subsequently in 1991, the Nadler group reported that IFNγ induces the transcription and expression of B7 molecules on the cell surface of monocytes, and speculated that this might be an additional mechanism whereby APCs might function to provide costimulatory signals via the B7/CD28 ligand/receptor system to productively activate T cells during an immune response.[14] In this regard, it is noteworthy that other known stimulants of monocytes/macrophages, such as M-CSF, GM-CSF, IL-3, TNFα, and LPS did not induce the expression of B7. Since IFNγ is produced by both T cells (both CD8+ and CD4+) and NK cells, with major effects on monocytes and macrophages, inducing their APC capacities, this represents a feed-forward system designed to maximally promote immune responses, both T cell-mediated as well as B cell-mediated.

Given that the B7/CD28 trigger serves as a co-stimulator together with TCR activation by pMHC, tumor immunologists wondered whether B7 expression by tumor cells could render non-immunogenic tumors to become immunogenic. Thus, in 1992 Linsley's group made use of a model system constructed of a murine melanoma that was transfected with the human papillomavirus-16 (HPV-16) E7 gene to ensure that the tumor cells expressed a tumor-specific antigen.[15] Even though expressing foreign antigens, these tumor cells grew pro-gressively in their hosts. However, as shown in 1995 transfection of these tumor cells with the gene encoding the costimulatory molecule B7 induced strong antitumor immunity to E7+ tumors, whether they expressed B7. Tumor rejection was T cell-mediated and B7-dependent, since treatment of mice with CTLA-4/Ig (see below) blocked rejection of E7+B7+ tumor cells. Also, inoculation of E7+B7- tumor-bearing mice with E7+B7+ tumor cells led to curative immunity against pro-gressively growing E7+B- micrometastases. The authors speculated that because of the ability to stimulate curative immunity, antitumor immune responses in cancer patients might be increased by stimulat-ing the T cell CD28 receptor. Similar findings were obtained using B7-2 in a different tumor cell system.[16]

CTLA-4, A Negative Feedback Molecule

While searching for genes selectively expressed by cytolytic T cells, in 1987 Pierre Golstein's group discovered a new member of the Ig superfamily encoding 223 amino acids.[17] The predicted primary struc-ture consisted of a single region homologous with an Ig V-region, and mRNA transcripts were only found in TCR-activated T cells. Golstein followed up this initial report in 1991 with a more detailed analysis of the CTLA-4 gene compared with the CD28 gene.[18] Both the mouse and human CTLA-4 and CD28 genes share the same overall intron/exon organization. Moreover, the nucleic acid sequence homology of the exons extends across both molecules and species. mRNA expression of human CTLA-4 was only detected in TCR/CD28-activated T cells. Finally, the CD28 and CTLA-4 genes map to the same chromosomal region in both the mouse and human, thereby suggesting that gene duplication had taken place.

Peter Linsley, working with Jeffrey Ledbetter's group in 1991 explored the functional significance of CTLA-4 by constructing a soluble CTLA-4/Ig fusion protein.[19] This genetically engineered gene product bound specifically to B7-transfected cells, as well as to B lymphoblastoid cells, and the fusion protein was capable of precipitating B7 from ^{125}I-labeled cell surface extracts. Most intriguing, the soluble CTLA-4-Ig fusion protein inhibited T cell proliferation in a mixed lymphocyte reaction (MLR), and helper T cell-induced Ig production by human B cells stimulated in an MLR. These findings thus supported the interpretation that CTLA-4 functioned as did CD28, as a co-stimulatory molecule for T cell activation.

In 1992, Linsley collaborated with Jeffrey Bluestone's group, exploring whether the CTLA-4/Ig fusion protein might also suppress immune responses *in vivo*.[20] They found that CTLA-4/Ig therapy blocked human pancreatic islet rejection in mice by directly affecting T cell recognition of B7+ APCs. In addition, CTLA-4/Ig induced long-term, donor-specific tolerance, prompting the investigators to speculate that this chimeric molecule might have uses to block rejection of human organ allo-transplantation. Simultaneously, Linsley and Ledbetter reported that CTLA-4/Ig suppressed T cell-dependent antibody responses to SRBC and Keyhole Limpet Hemocyanin (KLH), but did not induce tolerance to these very strong foreign antigens.[21] However, their results indicated that CTLA-4/Ig is capable of suppressing T cell-dependent humoral immune responses in addition to allogeneic T cell-mediated immune responses.

Interpreting experiments using the CTLA-4/Ig fusion molecule were limited, in that the exact mechanism whereby these molecules were inhibitory to immune responses remained obscure. However, in 1994 Craig Thompson and Jeffrey Bluestone collaborated with Peter Linsley and Gordon Freeman, and used a newly derived CTLA-4 reactive MoAb to perform additional functional experiments.[22] They found that stimulation of splenocytes with anti-CD3 promoted the expression of CTLA-4, but if they used CD28 (-/-) T cells,[23] CTLA-4 expression was markedly diminished on both CD4+ and CD8+ T cells. However, notably supplementation with rIL-2 at 50 U/mL largely reconstituted CTLA-4 expression of the CD28 (-/-) splenocytes, thereby indicating that CTLA-4 expression upon anti-CD3/CD28 activation is actually attributable to "signal 4," IL-2, rather than either the TCR ("signal 1") or CD28 ("signal 2") per se. Kinetic experiments revealed that, as noted by others, CTLA-4 expression was absent on resting cells, and first became detectable after 24 hours of stimulation with anti-CD3, peaking after 48 hours, to return to barely detectable levels by 96 hours of culture. In this regard, it is noteworthy that IL-2 production displays similar kinetics after mitogenic stimulation, which we had shown I 1978.[24]

Particularly noteworthy, functional assays, testing the effects of anti-CTLA-4 MoAbs revealed that there was a MoAb concentration-dependent *suppression* of T cell proliferation activated by either alloantigens in an MLR, or specific peptide-pMHC-induced proliferation of transgenic T cells. Thus, the anti-CTLA-4 MoAbs were not antagonistic but agonistic, and appeared to promote a *negative* signal mediated via CTLA-4. Of significance, they interpreted their results as showing that CTLA-4 normally functions to *suppress* IL-2 production. A year later in 1995 another anti-CTLA-4 MoAb was reported that yielded similar findings and conclusions.[25]

Accordingly, resting T cells first encounter APC-derived MHC-antigen complexes via their TCR in the presence of a co-stimulatory signal supplied by APC B7 to CD28. This interaction activates T cells to produce IL-2, which drives T cell proliferation and also activates CTLA-4 expression. At the time point of maximal CTLA-4 expression, B7/CD28 co-stimulatory function is diminished, because CTLA-4 preferentially ligates B7, as this interaction occurs with a 10–20-fold higher affinity compared with the B7/CD28 interaction.[22] Thus, CTLA-4 expression and function represents an *IL-2-induced negative feedback loop* that functions to attenuate the positive, pro-proliferation IL-2 signals via an inhibition of IL-2 production.

In 1995, two reports of CTLA-4 gene deleted mice appeared, one from Arlene Sharpe's group,[26] the other from Craig Thompson's group in collaboration with Tak Mak's group.[27] Both found that mice born without CTLA-4 expression rapidly developed lymphoproliferative disease with multi-organ lymphocytic infiltration and tissue destruction, with particularly severe myocarditis and pancreatitis. The mice became moribund and died by 3–4 weeks of age. Accordingly, these reports solidified the conclusion that CTLA-4 expressed on TCR/CD28-activated T cells normally functions as a negative regulator of T cell activation and is vital to circumvent systemic T cell-mediated multi-organ autoimmunity.

Maria-Luisa Alegre working in Craig Thompson's group subsequently provided definitive data in 1996 regarding the signals responsible for CTLA-4 expression, supporting an IL-2-induced negative feedback loop pivoting on CTLA-4. Employing anti-IL-2 and anti-IL-2R MoAbs, they found that almost all CTLA-4 expression was attributable to IL-2 after TCR activation. Then, using IL-2 (-/-) lymph node cells, which were deficient in CTLA-4 expression, they showed that supplementation with IL-2 overcame almost all of the deficient CTLA-4 expression. They interpreted the signals that promote CTLA-4 expression to be mostly due to IL-2, but they could not exclude signals emanating from either CD28 itself, or to other cytokines promoted by CD28 activation. The IL-2-induced, CTLA-4-mediated negative feedback loop was further substantiated by Mathew Krummel and James Allison, who reported in 1996 that CTLA-4 MoAb crosslinking, or binding to B7 on APCs, inhibited the production of IL-2.[28]

Dana Leach working with Krummel and Allison went one step further, also in 1996 asking whether anti-CTLA-4 MoAbs administered to tumor bearing mice could facilitate tumor rejection.[29] They utilized tumor cells transfected with B7-1, which Chen and co-workers had found previously[15,16] was successful in inducing tumor rejection. When mice were injected with anti-CTLA-4 MoAbs, there was *accelerated* rejection of B7-expressing tumors as compared with the mice injected either with anti-CD28 or no MoAbs. Of significance, the anti-CTLA-4 MoAb treatment worked even when administered therapeutically, after tumors were established, and the rejection resulted in immunity to a secondary exposure to the same tumor cells. They also observed these effects on unmanipulated wild-type tumors. It is noteworthy that there was no mention of a lymphoproliferative autoimmune syndrome developing in any of the mice that received the CTLA-4 blockade as anti-tumor therapy.

The Programmed Death (PD-1) Molecule, Another Negative Feedback Regulator

Searching for molecules that might be involved in activating programmed cell death pathways, in 1992 Tasuku Honjo's group used subtractive screening of a cDNA library made from a T cell line induced to undergo death by phorbol myristic acetate (PMA)/ionomycin and a library from a B cell line induced by anti-IgM.[30] These techniques resulted in the identification and isolation of a new member of the Ig superfamily with a single V-like external domain, which they termed Programmed Death-1 (PD-1). To provide data regarding function, in 1996 they developed a MoAb reactive with PD-1 that immunoprecipitated a 50–55 kDa membrane glycoprotein.[31] Expression of PD-1 membrane protein was limited to a small number of murine thymocytes, as well as splenocytes, lymph node cells and bone marrow cells, but within 48 hours after the administration of anti-CD3 MoAb, which resulted in massive cell death (75–95%) of the CD4+CD8+ "double positive" thymocytes, the remaining single positive thymocytes as well as the double negative thymocytes were found to be PD-1[+]. After anti-CD3 *in vitro* activation of either thymocytes or splenocytes there was a marked induction of PD-1 on T cells that peaked later, after 48–72 hours of culture, thus late after activation, very similar to CTLA-4 expression. The PD-1+ cells were large blastoid cells that co-expressed the activation markers IL-2Rα chain and CD69. Also, anti-IgM but not LPS, activated expression of PD-1 on splenic B cells.

The Honjo group went on to generate PD-1 gene-deleted mice in 1998 to further investigate the function of PD-1.[32] In marked contrast to CTLA-4 (-/-) mice, which became moribund and died between 3–4 weeks of age, PD-1 (-/-) mice on a C57Bl/6 background grew normally and appeared healthy. Even so, when examined at maturity, 6-weeks of age, there was noticeable splenomegaly, with a doubling of spleen weight and cell number, with ~40–50% increase in B cells and T cells, and a marked (~4-fold) increase in macrophages. Also significant, there were normal CD4+/CD8+ ratios in the spleens of the PD-1 (-/-) mice. When activated *in vitro* by anti-CD3, T cells from PD-1 (-/-) mice proliferated normally, while B cells activated with anti-IgM incorporated ~ twice the amounts of ^{3}H-Tdr. Measurement of serum Ig levels also pointed to an abnormality in the B cell compartment, in that IgG3 levels of PD-1 (-/-) mice were elevated compared with littermate control mice. Subsequent studies reported in 1999 on these B6 PD-1 (-/-) mice allowed to age beyond 6 weeks, revealed that at 6-months and 14-months of age the mice developed a systemic lupus-like syndrome, manifested by proliferative glomerulonephritis and rheumatoid-like arthritis.[33] Thus, it appeared that PD-1, like CTLA-4, normally functions to deliver a negative regulatory signal, but that the PD-1 signal was both qualitatively and quantitatively different from the CTLA-4 signal.

Search for a ligand reactive with PD-1 came to fruition in 2000. Gordon Freeman, Andrew Long and Yoshiko Iwai collaborated to identify a new member of the B7 molecular family, Programmed Death Ligand-1 (PDL-1), via a B-7 homology-based search of Expressed Sequence Tag (EST) databases.[34] PDL-1 is expressed by APCs, including INFγ-stimulated human monocytes and murine dendritic cells (DCs). Also, noteworthy was the finding that PDL-1 is expressed by non-lymphoid tissues, such as heart and lung. Ligation of PD-1 by PDL-1 results in inhibition of TCR-mediated cytokine production and subsequent proliferation, especially if the T cell stimuli, either anti-CD3 or anti-CD28, are suboptimal.

Continuing their quest to discover PD-1 functions, in 2001 Hiroyki Nishimura and co-workers from the Honjo group bred the PD-1 (-/-) onto the Balb/c background.[35] In sharp contrast to the B6 PD-1 (-/-) strain, the Balb/c PD-1 (-/-) mice started to die as early as 5 weeks of age, and by 30 weeks, 2/3 of the mice had succumbed. That this premature mortality was secondary to an immunological phenomenon was supported by the fact that Balb/c-PD-1 (-/-)-RAG2 (-/-) mice survived normally. The accelerated mortality was ascribed to dilated cardiomyopathy with severely impaired cardiac contractility and sudden death by congestive heart failure. Affected hearts were found to have diffuse deposition of IgG on the surface of the cardiomyocytes, and all the affected PD-1 (-/-) mice had high titer circulating IgG autoantibodies reactive with a 33 kDa protein on the surface of cardiomyocytes, indicating that this was a humoral autoimmune reaction. In this regard, they did not find a diffuse infiltration of inflammatory cells into the myocardium, so that this cardiac abnormality was distinct from the T cell-mediated cardiomyositis seen in the CTLA-4 (-/-) mice.

Concomitantly in 2001, Gordon Freeman in collaboration with Honjo's group, as well as Beatriz Carreno and Laura Carter, reported the discovery of a second PD-1 ligand, PD-L2.[36] GENBANK was searched, looking for PD-L1 homologs, and ultimately both murine and human cDNAs were identified that predicted 70% amino acid identity. Like the other members of the B7 family, PD-L2 shares a structural organization consisting of a signal sequence, followed by an Ig-V-like, IgC-like, transmembrane and short cytoplasmic domains. Comparison of PD-L1 and PD-L2 mRNA expression revealed that they were similar in normal tissues, with high expression in placenta, and low expression in spleen, lymph nodes and thymus. Both mRNAs were expressed in human heart, but some tissues, such as human pancreas, lung and liver expressed PD-L2 but not PD-L1. Like PD-L1, PD-L2 expression was undetectable on normal human monocytes, but could be induced by IFNγ. The two ligands are also functionally similar, in that they both dampen anti-CD3-promoted T cell cytokine production and proliferation. Accordingly, the investigators speculated that the PD-1/PD-L pathway may play a key role in the induction and/or maintenance of peripheral tolerance and autoimmune diseases. Also, because PD-L1 and PD-L2 can inhibit effector T cell cytokine production and proliferation, it was speculated that the pathway could serve as an attractive therapeutic target, in that blocking the pathway could enhance immune reactivity, for example against cancer, whereas stimulating this pathway could be useful to attenuating ongoing immune responses, such as in transplant rejection, autoimmune and allergic diseases.

In this regard, in 2002 Laura Carter and Beatriz Carreno collaborated again with the Freeman and Honjo groups to examine the mechanism responsible for PD-1/PD-L inhibition of T cell activation, and concluded that proliferation is inhibited as a result of compromised IL-2 production.[37] T cells stimulated with anti-CD3+ PD-L1-coated beads display dramatically decreased IL-2 production and resultant proliferation, while CFSE analysis showed fewer cycling cells and a slower division rate. Moreover, both CD4+ and CD8+ cells are susceptible to this inhibitory pathway. However noteworthy, exogenous IL-2 was able to circumvent PD-L1-mediated inhibition, indicating that the activated cells maintain IL-2 responsiveness.

Carreno and co-workers followed up in 2003 with a further analysis of the effects of PD-1 activation on human T cell cytokine production.[38] First, of significance they showed that after anti-CD3 stimulation of purified, macrophage-depleted T cells most CD4+ T cells express both PD-L1 and PD-L2, a distinct difference from CTLA-4 and its ligands, B7-1 and B7-2, which are expressed by APCs, but not expressed by the T cells themselves. Second, they found that PD-1-mediated inhibition of cytokine production and proliferation overrides ICOS (another costimulatory molecule) co-stimulation of purified T cells but not CD28 costimulation, an effect that they found due to the low concentrations of IL-2 produced by ICOS vs. CD28 co-stimulation. Moreover, cytokines that activate STAT5, such as IL-2, IL-7 and IL-15, were capable of overcoming the PD-1 inhibition, whereas other cytokines that act as T cell growth factors but activate other STATs, such as IL-4 (STAT6) and IL-21 (STAT1 & STAT3), could not. Since IL-2 is only produced by TCR-activated T cells, while IL-7 and IL-15 are produced by stromal cells, these findings underscore the key role of *T cell IL-2-induced negative feedback loops* in regulating the tempo, magnitude and duration of IL-2 promoted T cell immune responses.

References

1. Hansen J, Martin P, and Nowinski R. (1980). Monoclonal antibodies identifying a novel T cell antigen and Ia antigens of human lymphocytes. *Immunogenetics* **10**:247–260.

2. Lum L, Orcutt-Thordarson N, Seigneuret M, and Hansen J. (1982). *In vitro* regulation of immunoglobulin synthesis by T cell subpopulations defined by a new human T cell antigen. *Cell Immunol* **72**:122–129.
3. Ledbetter J, Martin P, Spooner C, *et al.* (1985). Antibodies to Tp67 and Tp44 augment and sustain proliferative reponses of activated T cells. *J Immunol* **135**:2331–2336.
4. Aruffo A and Seed B. (1987). Molecular cloning of a CD28 cDNA by high efficiency COS cell expression system. *Proc Natl Acad Sci USA* **84**:8573–8577.
5. Thompson C, Lindstrom T, Ledbetter J, *et al.* (1989). CD28 activation pathway regulates the production of multiple T cell-derived lymphokines/cytokines. *J Immunol* **86**:1333–1337.
6. Lindsten T, June C, Ledbetter J, *et al.* (1989). Regulation of lymphokine messanger RNA stability by a surface-mediated T cell activation pathway. *Science* **244**:339–343.
7. Fraser JD, Irving BA, Crabtree GR, and Weiss A. (1991). Regulation of interleukin-2 gene enhancer activity by the T cell accessory molecule CD28. *Science* **251**:313–316.
8. Ghosh P, Tan T-H, Rice NR, Sica A, and Young HA. (1993). The interleukin 2 CD28-responsive complex contains at least three members of the NF-kB family: c-Rel, p50, and p65. *Proc Natl Acad Sci USA* **90**:1696–1700.
9. Garrity PA, Chen D, Rothenberg EV, and Wold BJ. (1994). Interleukin 2 transcription is regulated *in vivo* at the level of coordinated binding of both constitutive and regulated factors. *Mol Cell Bio* **14**:2159–2169.
10. Rothenberg EV and Ward SB. (1996). A dynamic assembly of diverse transcription factors integrates activation and cell-type information for interleukin 2 gene regulation. *Proc Natl Acad Sci USA* **93**:9358–9365.
11. Liou H, Jin Z, Tumang J, *et al.* (1999). c-Rel is crucial for lymphocyte proliferation but dispensable for T cell effector function. *Int Immunol* **11**:361–371.
12. Freedman A, Freeman G, Horowitz J, *et al.* (1987). B7, a B cell-restricted antigen that identifies preactivated B cells. *J Immunol* **139**:3260–3267.
13. Freeman G, Freedman A, Segil J, *et al.* (1989). B7, a new member of the IG superfamily with unique expression on activated and neoplastic B cells. *J Immunol* **143**:2714–2722.
14. Freedman A, Freeman G, Rhynhart K, and Nadler L. (1991). Selective induction of B7/BB-1 on interferon-gamma stimulated monocytes: A potential mechanism for amplification of T cell activation through the CD28 pathway. *Cell Immunol* **137**:429–437.

15. Chen L, Ashe S, Brady W, et al. (1992). Costimulation of antitumor immunity by the B7 counterreceptor for the T lymphocyte molecules CD28 and CTLA-4. *Cell* **71**:1093–1102.

16. Yang G, Hellstrom K, Hellstrom I, and Chen L. (1995). Antitumor immunity elicited by tumor cells transfected with B7-2, a second ligand for CD28/CTLA-4 costimunatory molecules. *J Immunol* **154**:2794–2800.

17. Brunet J, Denizot F, Luciani M, et al. (1987). A new member of the immunoglobulin superfamily-CTLA-4. *Nature* **328**:267–270.

18. Harper K, Balzano C, Rouvier E, et al. (1991). CTLA-4 and CD28 activated lymphocyte molecules are closely related in both mouse and human as to sequence, message expression, gene structure, and chromosomal location. *J Immunol* **147**:1037–1044.

19. Linsley P, Brady W, Urnes M, et al. (1991). CTLA-4 is a second receptor for the B cell activation antigen B7. *J Exp Med* **174**:561–569.

20. Lenschow D, Zeng Y, Thistlewaite J, et al. (1992). Long-term survival of xenogeneic pancreatic islet grafts induced by CTLA-4Ig. *Science* **257**:789–792.

21. Linsley P, Wallace P, Johnson J, et al. (1992). Immunosuppression *in vivo* by a soluble form of the CTLA-4/Ig T cell activation molecule. *Science* **257**:792–795.

22. Walunas T, Lenschow D, Bakker C, et al. (1994). CTLA-4 can function as a negative regulator of T cell activation. *Immunity* **1**:405–413.

23. Shahinian A, Pfeffer K, Lee K, et al. (1993). Differential T cell costimulation requirements in CD-28-deficient mice. *Science* **261**:609–612.

24. Gillis S, Ferm MM, Ou W, and Smith KA. (1978). T cell growth factor: Parameters of production and a quantitative microassay for activity. *J Immunol* **120**:2027–2032.

25. Krummel M and Allison J. (1995). CD28 and CTLA-4 have opposing effects on the response of T cells to stimulation. *J Exp Med* **182**:459–465.

26. Tivol E, Borriello F, Schweitzer A, et al. (1995). Loss of CTLA-4 leads to massive lymphoproliferation and fatal multiorgan tissue destruction, revealing c critical negative regulatory role of CTLA-4. *Immunity* **3**:541–547.

27. Waterhouse P, Penningger J, Timms E, et al. (1995). Lymphoproliferative disorders with early lethality in mice deficient in CTLA-4. *Science* **270**:985–988.

28. Krummel M and Allison J. (1996). CTLA-4 engagement inhibits IL-2 accumulation and cell cycle progression upon activation of resting T cells. *J Exp Med* **183**:2533–2540.

29. Leach D, Krummel M, and Allison J. (1996). Enhancement of antitumor immunity by CTLA-4 blockade. *Science* **271**:1734–1736.

30. Ishida Y, Agata Y, Shibahara K, and Honjo, T. (1992). Induced expression of PD-1, a novel member of the immunoglobulin gene superfamily, upon programmed cell death. *EMBO J* **11**:3887–3895.

31. Agata Y, Kawasaki A, Nishimura H, *et al.* 1996. Expression of th PD-1 antigen on the surface of stimulated mouse and B lymphocytes. *Int Immunol* **8**:765–772.

32. Nishimura H, Minato N, Nakano T, and Honjo T. (1998). Immunological studies on PD-1-deficient mice: Implication of PD-1 as a negative regulator for B cell responses. *Int Immunol* **10**:1563–1572.

33. Nishimura H, Nose M, Hiai H, *et al.* (1999). Development of lupus-like autoimmune diseases by disruption of the PD-1 gene encoding an ITIM motif-carrying immunoreceptor. *Immunity* **11**:141–151.

34. Freeman G, Long A, Iwai Y, *et al.* (2000). Engagement of the PD-1 immunoinhibitory receptor by a novel B7 family member leads to negative regulation of lymphocyte activation. *J Exp Med* **192**:1027–1034.

35. Nishimura H, Okazaki T, Tanaka Y, *et al.* (2001). Autoimmune dilated cardiomyopathy in PD-1 receptor-deficient mice. *Science* **291**:319–322.

36. Latchman Y, Wood CR, Chernova T, *et al.* (2001). PD-L2 is a second ligand for PD-1 and inhibits T cell activation. *Nat Immunol* **2**:261–268.

37. Carter L, Fouser L, Jussif J, *et al.* (2002). PD-1:PDL inhibitory pathway affects both CD4+ and CD8+ T cells and is overcome by IL2. *Eur J Immunol* **32**:634–643.

38. Bennett F, Luxenberg D, Ling V, *et al.* (2003). Program death-1 engagement upon TCR activation has distinct effects on costimulation and cytokine-driven proliferation: Attenuation of ICOS, IL-4, and IL-21, but not CD28, IL-7, and IL-15 responses. *J Immunol* **170**:711–718.

8 Regulatory T Cells

The Origin of "Regulatory" Cells

In the 1960s, Jacques Miller became focused on uncovering the function of the thymus soon after the realization that there were two arms of the system, the humoral and the cell-mediated arm. At this time, the thymus was regarded as enigmatic. Histologically, the thymus was comprised of small, apparently well differentiated small lymphocytes, but if the thymus was removed there was no apparent effect on immunological function. Thus, the immunological cognoscenti concluded that there was no special functional role for the thymus, apparently thinking that the thymus was simply a storehouse for mature lymphocytes. Miller resisted this notion, and so he went further, devising methods to thymectomize newborn mice, speculating that the thymus might play some role in the development of the immune system. In 1961 he published the first of a series of articles detailing the effects of neonatal thymectomy within the first three days of life, which became termed day three thymectomy (d3Tx).[1,2] For the first four weeks of life, d3Tx mice appeared grossly normal and grew identically with sham thymectomized control mice. However, over the next several weeks in the second month of life, the d3Tx mice failed to thrive and lost weight, becoming runted, like mice with Graft vs. Host (GvH) disease, and died prematurely from a syndrome characterized by wasting and diarrhea.

Miller studied the immunological reactivity of d3Tx mice and found that even though the mice appeared normal in the first few weeks of life, actually the mice were markedly immunocompromized, manifested by severe lymphopenia of primary and secondary lymphoid organs, an inability to mount an antibody response when immunized, and an incapacity to reject both allogeneic and even xenogeneic skin grafts. Therefore, there was an immunodeficiency of both the humoral and cell-mediated immune systems. Even so, later when the mice became runted in the second month of life with GvH-like disease, there was a marked infiltration of many organs by activated lymphocytes, and Miller emphasized this point, although he was most interested in the earlier immunodeficiency. These reports by Miller were the first exposition of the paradox of hyperimmune reactivity and systemic autoimmunity coexisting with immunodeficiency.

Miller's observations concerning this paradoxical hyper-autoimmunity and immunodeficiency went unexplored for 20 years until 1982, when Shimon Sakaguchi and co-workers reported that d3Tx mice, as well as athymic *(nu/nu)* mice, would develop autoimmune inflammation in multiple organs, including oophoritis, gastritis, thyroiditis, and orchitis when reconstituted with normal adult T cells lacking the Lyt-1+ subset of cells.[3] Until this time, the Lyt-1 alloantigen was thought to distinguish the Th subset from the cytolytic T cell subset, based on cytolytic assays using alloantisera reactive with Lyt-1 and Lyt-2/3 + C'.[4] However, Len Herzenberg's group had reported in 1980 using the more sensitive flow cytometer and immunofluorescence that Lyt-1 was expressed by all T cells in varying densities.[5] Nonetheless, Sakaguchi postulated that removing the thymus early in life before the immune system had developed completely might result in deprivation of a critical subset of T cells that normally might function to *"suppress or regulate"* potential self-reactive T cell clones, a phenomenon now termed central tolerance. In an accompanying report, Sakaguchi went on to show that *nu/nu* mice or d3Tx mice reconstituted with Lyt-1+ T cells could prevent the development of the severe autoimmune disorders.[6] In these two publications, Sakaguchi first speculated that the depletion of this *"regulatory T cell"* subset by d3Tx might result in the post-thymectomy autoimmune diseases. He then confirmed these observations by another publication in 1985.[7]

The IL-2 (-/-) Mouse: Immunodeficient and Autoimmune

The IL-2 gene was the first cytokine gene to be deleted, reported by Ivan Horak and co-workers in 1991.[8] Since IL-2 was considered essential for proliferative clonal expansion of antigen-activated T cells, it was anticipated that IL-2 gene deletion would result in severe T cell immunodeficiency. The results of the first experiments reported were intriguing. IL-2 (-/-) mice appeared normal at birth, with no evidence of lymphopenia or immunodeficiency. However, *in vitro* experiments performed with splenocytes from young mice did show the expected deficiencies, in that proliferative responses to mitogens such as ConA were decreased by ~70% compared to littermate controls. Even so, Horak's team were surprised to find any residual proliferative activity from the IL-2 (-/-) T cells at all, given the newly established dogma that mitogenic T cell proliferative responses are mitogen- or antigen-activated but IL-2-mediated.

To further characterize the immunological status of IL-2 (-/-) mice in 1993, Horak collaborated with Hans Hengartner and Rolf Zinkernagel, who were well versed in microbial infectious disease models in mice. Thus, when challenged with the viral pathogens Lymphocytic Chorio-Meningitis Virus (LCMV) or Vesicular Stomatitis Virus (VSV), the IL-2 (-/-) mice were immunocompromized compared with controls, but again, immune responses were not totally absent.[9] The generation of CTL reactivity was found to be 1/3 of the control mice, and the IL-2 (-/-) mice recovered from their infections instead of succumbing. These investigators interpreted their results as, "these *normal in vivo* immune responses question the importance of IL-2 as defined by *in vitro* studies."

One explanation of these findings was that cytokines were redundant and that other cytokines could substitute for IL-2, either IL-4, or even other cytokines yet to be discovered. Two years later, in 1995 Christine Biron's group made a more thorough study of IL-2 (-/-) mice infected with LCMV.[10] They found that the robust proliferative expansion of LCMV-specific CTL was virtually absent in IL-2 (-/-) mice and the generation of CTL activity was depressed by 90% compared with controls. Thus, all of these experiments essentially reinforced the role of IL-2 as an important T cell-derived hormone for an efficient robust T cell immune response.

Subsequently however, when the IL-2 (-/-) mice were allowed to age beyond puberty at 5–6 weeks, a paradoxical polyclonal lymphoproliferative autoimmune syndrome was reported in 1995 by

Horak and co-workers.[11] Moreover, when the IL-2 gene deletion was bred to a Balb/c background, the autoimmune lymphoproliferative disease was accelerated, with almost 100% mortality by 5 weeks of age. Remarkably similar to GvH disease, activated T cells were found invading multiple organs, including salivary glands, lungs, kidneys, heart, pancreas and liver. Furthermore, autoimmune hemolytic anemia and inflammatory bowel disease eventually led to premature death. Although both CD4+ and CD8+ T cells became activated, as detected by morphology and activation surface markers like CD44 and CD69, the appearance of activated CD4+ T cells preceded CD8+ T cells and B cells. In 1995, these findings led us to the hypothesis that an unanticipated crucial defect resulting from IL-2 deficiency might be the absence of the development of an IL-2-dependent *negative feedback* pathway.[12]

The *Scurfy* Mouse

In 1949, a spontaneous mutation was noted in a mouse colony at the Oak Ridge Tennessee National Laboratory. The mutation was propagated and reported by geneticists William and Lianne Russell in 1959 to be X-linked and recessive, leading to a failure to thrive syndrome in males, manifested by ruffled fur and weight loss.[13] Male *scurfy* mice suffered from an autoimmune lymphoproliferative syndrome, which was very acute in onset soon after birth, leading to death by 3 weeks of age. The macroscopic appearance of the mice included runting, scaly skin, squinted eyes, hepatosplenomegally, and lymphadenopathy. Characteristic histological findings included a lymphohistiocytic proliferation and infiltration that destroyed normal lymph node architecture, thickened the dermis, with nodular germinal center-like accumulations in the hepatic portal areas.[14] Also, a severe autoimmune hemolytic anemia occurred together with a marked polyclonal gammopathy. Thus, this syndrome was very similar to the runting, GvH-like syndrome suffered by the d3Tx mice of Miller, and those lymphopenic immunodeficient *nu/nu* or d3Tx mice reconsitituted with adult T cells lacking Lyt1+ T cells, as well as the IL-2 (-/-) and CTLA-4 (-/-) mice. Most important, scurfy heterozygous females (i.e. X^{sf}/X^+), with 50%

of their T cells containing the mutant gene and 50% containing the normal gene, were entirely normal, thereby suggesting that the normal T cells could somehow suppress the T cells carrying the mutant gene from becoming hyperactive.

It took more than 30 years for the field of immunology to mature to the point that cellular and molecular analyses of the immunological defects of these mice were possible. In a series of reports beginning in 1991, Virginia Godfrey, working with J. Erby Wilkinson and Lianne Russell, demonstrated that the scurfy phenotype was attributable to an abnormality primarily but not entirely of CD4+ T cells.[15-17] Thus, treatment of mice with MoAbs to remove CD8+ T cells neither lessened the severity of the disease nor changed the acute disease onset, whereas removal of CD4+ T cells alleviated the severity of the lesions and significantly increased lifespan. Although fairly normal at 3 weeks of age, CD4-deficient scurfy mice begin exhibiting signs of scurfy disease at four weeks, including enlarged lymph nodes, splenomegaly, activated T and B cell areas in lymphoid organs, elevated serum IgG levels, with death by ~6 weeks of age. Thus, their lifespan is only doubled when CD4+ T cells are absent.

Focusing on potential molecular mechanisms of scurfy disease, in 1996 Godfrey, Wilkinson and others revealed an over-expression of cytokine genes.[17] Using northern blots, quantitative PCR and in situ hybridization, these investigators found increased expression of IL-2, IL-4, IL-5, IL-6, IL-7, IL-10, IFNγ and TNFα. Further experiments found increased production of GM-CSF and Mac1+ cells, as well overexpression of co-stimulatory ligands, B7-1 and B7-2 by APCs. Most significant, like CTLA4 (-/-) T cells, scurfy T cells proliferated in vitro without TCR stimulation and had a decreased requirement for co-stimulation. Thus, all together these findings provided a molecular basis for the inflammatory pathology characteristic of the scurfy phenotype, and were consistent with the interpretation that the scurfy mutation yields a loss of function of a "normal down-regulation of T cell activation." Given the striking resemblance of the scurfy phenotype with the d3Tx phenotype, the CTLA-4 (-/-) phenotype and the IL-2 (-/-) phenotype, the fact that the scurfy CD4+ T cells expressed the IL-2Rα chain, as well as other activation markers such as CD69, suggested that all four of these abnormal double immuno-deficient/autoimmune mice could very well be attributed to a common molecular mechanism.

T-Regs and the IL-2Rα Chain

Also in 1995, a decade after Sakaguchi initially coined the term "regulatory T cell," his group followed up his initial reports, this time showing that lymphopenic *nu/nu* mice developed a lethal lymphoproliferative syndrome if reconstituted with adult T cells from which IL-2Rα⁺ T cells had been removed.[18] Moreover, the subset of normal adult T cells that expressed the IL-2Rα chain (<10%), usually thought of as a marker for antigen-activated T cells, prevented the development of the multi-organ autoimmune disease, which included thyroiditis, gastritis, insulinitis, sialoadenitis, adrenalitis, oophoritis, glomerulonephritis, and polyarthritis. Thus began an explosion of research into regulatory T cells, termed T-Regs.

Early on in this research, the only way to identify T-Regs was the expression of the IL-2Rα chain. However, in this regard, it warrants particular emphasis that although most of the IL-2Rα⁺ T cells were also CD4⁺, Sakaguchi found that CD8⁺ T cells that express the IL-2Rα chain were also effective in preventing the autoimmune syndrome. Sakaguchi followed up these reports with similar experiments in 1996 using d3Tx mice as recipients of various T cell subsets.[19] Also, they established that IL2-Rα⁺ T cells were undetectable at birth, first became detectable in the periphery after day 3 in the neonatal period, and reached adult levels by two weeks after birth, with ~10% of splenocyte CD4⁺ T cells and < 1% CD8⁺ T cells becoming IL2-Rα⁺, presumably as a consequence of antigen activation in the first days of postnatal life. Thus established, they then found that d3Tx retards the accumulation of splenic T cells by 90%, and that IL2-Rα⁺ T cells were essentially undetectable, thereby confirming Miller's report of 30 years earlier that d3Tx mice are T cell lymphopenic, but now with the additional observation that they did not develop IL2-Rα⁺ T cells.

Obviously, the difficulty with using the IL2-Rα chain as a marker for T-Regs resided with the fact that antigen activated T cells would also be found within this subset. When tested, adult IL2-Rα⁺ T cells expressed transcripts for IL2-Rα chain, IL-2, IL-4, IL-10, and IFNγ, consistent with this notion. Even so, it was hypothesized that the peripheral T cell population of d3Tx mice must have contained some self-reactive T cells, but insufficient numbers of IL2-Rα⁺ T-Regs to control or inhibit the self-reactive cells. In support of this hypothesis, there was clearly a dose-effect of the IL2-Rα⁺ cells, when tested to prevent gastritis of d3Tx mice. However, again it is noteworthy that CD8⁺ IL2-Rα⁺ T cells were also protective in this model, so that the investigators were very careful not to designate whether the T-Reg cells were derived from the CD4⁺ or the CD8⁺ T cell subsets, thereby implicating IL-2 and the IL-2Rα chain as the critical molecules involved in this phenomenon.

Do T-Regs "Suppress" Autoreactive T cells?

The model used by Sakaguchi to study this phenomenon was the lymphopenic mouse, either adult *nu/nu* or neonatal d3Tx mice. Thus, the paradox was how lymphopenia, which results in immunodeficiency, could evolve into lymphoproliferation to the point of self-reactivity. Obviously, these phenomena were at the heart of self/non-self recognition and tolerance, especially peripheral tolerance. However, the use of the *in vivo* systems was cumbersome when trying to elucidate mechanisms was concerned, so that there was a need for an *in vitro* system to study the suppressive phenomenon. Ethan Shevach's group developed such a system in 1998, using normal adult IL-2Rα-CD4⁺ T cells as target cells, mixed with a source of APCs (T cell-depleted irradiated splenocytes) as "accessory cells," and the whole mixture was activated with suboptimal concentrations of anti-CD3 (0.5 μg/mL).[20,21]

When IL-2Rα⁺ "T-Reg" cells from normal adult mice were mixed with the IL-2Rα- target cells at high T-Reg cell percentages (i.e. 50% to 12.5% T-Regs) a T-Reg cell concentration-dependent inhibition of tritiated thymidine (³H-TdR) incorporation was observed. However, if diluted beyond these high T-Reg cell percentages, to <10%, the inhibitory effect disappeared. In this regard, it is important to note that unfractionated splenocytes from normal adult mice normally contain ~ 10% IL-2Rα⁺ T cells, and they proliferate unimpeded under these circumstances. Also, it is worthy of emphasis that Shevach stressed that the non-T, accessory cells were necessary to observe the suppressive effect.

Using this polyclonal T cell proliferation assay, in 1998 Angela Thornton and Shevach made the following claims[21]: (1) normal adult purified IL-2Rα⁺ are anergic, in that they fail to proliferate in response to stimulation via anti-CD3, (2) IL-2Rα⁺ T cells markedly suppress the proliferation of anti-CD3-activated IL-2Rα-T cells by specifically inhibiting the production of IL-2, (3) the inhibition requires close contact between the suppressor cells and the responder cells and is not cytokine-mediated, (4) The inhibition requires activation of the "suppressor cells" via the TCR, (5) inhibition can be overcome by IL-2 or anti-CD28, suggesting that the suppressor cells block a co-stimulatory signal, such as CD28, and (6) induction of IL-2Rα expression *in vitro* or *in vivo* does not result in suppressive activity. Thus, these investigators concluded that IL-2Rα⁺CD4⁺T cells are present in normal mice, and represent "*a distinct lineage of "professional" suppressor cells.*"

FOXP3, the Gene Responsible for XLAAD, IPEX and the Scurfy (*sf*) Phenotype

In 2001, the fields of human primary immunodeficiencies and murine genetics converged. Fred Ramsdell's group, in collaboration with Wilkinson's group, which had originally identified the (*sf*) mutation, found a frame-shift mutation in the gene encoding FOXP3, a new member of the forkhead/winged-helix family of transcriptional regulators.[22] Coincident with this report, the human FOXP3 gene was found mutated in individuals suffering from the X-linked autoimmunity-allergic dysregulation (XLAAD) syndrome,[23] as well as the X-linked, neonatal diabetes mellitus, enteropathy and polyendocrinopathy (IPEX) syndrome by Ramsdell and others.[24,25] Thus, these reports established the unique function of the FOXP3 gene and its product for normal immunological homeostasis. Like the *scurfy* mice, individuals with mutant FOXP3 suffer from severe autoimmunity with rapid death. Also, just like mutants of CTLA-4, PD-1, and IL-2, mutations in the FOXP3 gene appeared to markedly derange the capacity of the immune system to remain quiescent when confronted with autoantigens, so that they lost self/nonself discrimination. Accordingly, these data pointed to a mechanistic relationship of these genes and their products as the keys to the paradoxical mingling of autoimmunity and immunodeficiency.

Also in 2001, experiments directed toward understanding FOXP3 function in the immune system revealed that the forkhead domain of the gene product is required for nuclear localization and DNA binding.[26] Moreover, upon over-expression in CD4+ T cells, FOXP3 inhibits the transcription of NF-AT response elements from the IL-2 promoter thereby attenuating TCR-activation of IL-2 production. Thus, this finding is consistent with the observations of hyperactive cytokine production from TCR-activated *scurfy* T cells, in that mutational crippling of this negative feedback loop, would lower the threshold of TCR signals required for IL-2 gene expression, and other cytokine genes as well. These data lead to the inevitable conclusion that FOXP3 constitutes another negative feedback loop that down-regulates TCR-activated cytokine gene expression. However, in contrast to CTLA-4 and PD-1, which interfere with TCR complex signaling at the level of the membrane, FOXP3 interferes with IL-2 transcription. Removal of any of these negative feedback loops would necessarily result in a chronic over production of IL-2 and other cytokine genes.

Although loss of function mutations of the genes encoding each of these molecules (i.e. IL-2, FOXP3, CTLA-4, PD-1) results in a similar systemic autoimmune pathologic syndrome, it was not clear whether these molecules were linked functionally. The kinetics of the onset of the autoimmune syndromes differed, in that IL-2 (-/-) mice resembled d3Tx mice, with a delayed onset of T cell proliferation and organ invasion after the 1st month of life. By comparison, CTLA-4 (-/-) mice succumbed rapidly, within the 1st month of life, while PD-1 (-/-) mice did not even develop a T lymphoproliferative syndrome, but rather a slow onset of antibody-mediated myocardial dysfunction, depending on the strain of mice used. However, those investigators interested in T-Reg cells recognized the striking similarities between the syndromes suffered by the FOXP3 (*scurfy*) mutants and the autoimmune syndrome of lymphopenic mice reconstituted with T cells lacking IL-2Rα chains. Accordingly, three simultaneous reports in 2003 (from Sakaguchi, Rudensky and Ramsdell) revealed that FOXP3 expression is restricted primarily to CD4+IL-2Rα+ cells.[27–29] Furthermore, each of these reports showed that cells with this phenotype were capable of suppressing T cell proliferation *in vitro*.

The Molecular Mechanism(s) of T-Reg Suppression

Because the T-Reg phenotype accepted by most investigators solidified around CD4+IL-2Rα+CTLA-4+FOXP3+, after 2003 investigators began probing for molecular explanations of the remarkable suppressive capacity of these cells. One simple explanation forwarded early on was that because of the high density expression of the IL-2Rα chains, perhaps these cells simply competed with the effector T cells (T_{eff}) for IL-2. T-Reg cells express not only a high density of the IL-2Rα chains but also IL-2Rβ and γ chains, which are required to signal rapid IL-2 internalization and degradation.[30] In 2007 Pushpa Pandiyan, working in Michael Lenardo's lab, examined this hypothesis in detail, and found that indeed T-Reg cells rapidly deplete IL-2, eventually leading to cytokine deprivation-induced cell death.[31]

Onar Feinerman, working in Gregoire Altan-Bonnet's group and collaborating with me then provided the molecular mechanisms responsible for the voracious IL-2 consumptive capacity of T-Regs in a series of experiments reported in 2010.[32] One rapid response to IL-2 signaling is a marked upregulation of IL-2Rα chain expression, as much as 20-fold, which was noted in our earliest experiments from 1985,[33] and now is known to be transmitted from the IL-2R to the IL-2Rα gene promoters by STAT5.[34] When monitored experimentally by Feinerman, extremely low IL-2 concentrations, e.g. 60 fM, attributable to an increase in affinity of the IL-2R due the high density of IL-2Rα chains, rapidly induce a further increase of IL-2Rα chain expression by T-Reg cells. This provides a feed-forward mechanism driving T-Reg cells to bind, internalize and degrade IL-2 at the expense of T_{eff}. And because FOXP3 is an IL-2-induced gene product that not only negatively regulates IL-2 gene expression by the T-Reg cells themselves, but activates expression of IL-2Rα chains, thereby favoring the rapid depletion of IL-2 from the milieu, this represents an exquisite IL-2-induced negative feedback loop that prevents IL-2-promoted expansion of antigen-triggered T_{eff} cells, particularly when only low IL-2 concentrations are available. Thus, T-Reg cells act as dominant-negative regulators, scavenging any IL-2 produced by T_{eff} cells within their vicinity.

CTLA-4 is the other phenotypic marker expressed by T-Reg cells. In this regard, it is important to note that CTLA-4 is constitutively expressed by T-Reg cells, but is dependent upon IL-2 activation of TCR-triggered T_{eff} cells (ergo, it's name of Cytolytic T cell Late Activation molecule) for their optimal expression as shown by Marie Louise Alegre in 1996.[35] To discriminate between the relative roles of CTLA-4 expressed by IL-2-activated T_{eff} cells and T-Reg cells in the rapid development of the terminal lymphoproliferative and autoimmune syndrome of CTLA-4 (-/-) mice, in 2004 Alegre's team followed up their earlier report, and tested the hypothesis that reduced expression of CTLA-4 in IL-2 (-/-) T cells in IL-2 (-/-) mice leads to their hyper-lymphoproliferative/autoimmune phenotype. Thus, expression of CTLA-4 as a transgene in IL-2 (-/-) mice completely prevented both lymphoaccumulation and autoimmune hemolytic anemia. Moreover, the effect of the CTLA-4 transgene was due to the expression of CTLA-4 on conventional T-cells rather than T-Reg cells.[36]

Then, four years later, in 2008 Kajsa Wing working in Shimon Sakaguchi's lab, examined directly the role of CTLA-4 in T-Reg suppressive function and showed that a T-Reg-specific CTLA-4 (-/-) results in spontaneous development of systemic lymphoproliferation, fatal T cell-mediated autoimmune disease, and of special note, also produces potent antitumor immunity.[37] They found that T-Reg-specific CTLA-4 deficiency impairs both *in vivo* and *in vitro* T-Reg suppressive function, especially the capacity of T-Regs to down-regulate CD80 and CD86 on dendritic cells, one of the major ways that T-Regs suppress activated T cell IL-2 production. Accordingly, T-Regs display at least three ways that combine to restrict IL-2 availability to antigen-activated T_{eff} cells, and thereby control the magnitude of T cell mediated immune responses.

Each of these gene deletion experiments were informative regarding the function of individual genes and their products in whole animals, but suffered a major drawback in that it was impossible to interpret the effects of gene deletion on embryogenesis and early development vs. the removal of a gene from a fully developed adult. Consequently, in 2016, Wing followed up her earlier report, using conditional CTLA-4 (-/-) mice to compare with germline congenital CTLA-4 deficiency.[38] Using the C57BL/10.Q strain, tamoxifen-inducible Cre was used to delete CTLA-4 from adult mice at 6–8 weeks of age (iKO), which was accomplished after three tamoxifen doses. Because germline CTLA-4 (-/-) mice succumb to the fatal lymphoproliferative syndrome before weaning (~30 days), iKO mice were first monitored for long-term survival and were found to survive beyond 100 days after CTLA-4 gene deletion. Even so, both iKO and cKO mice suffered massive lymphadenopathy and splenomegaly and hypergammaglobulinemia. Moreover, the iKO mice had substantial focal lymphocytic infiltration around the bronchioles, in the salivary glands and stomach, while notably heart and kidney remained unaffected. Also noteworthy, the lymphocytic infiltrates were comprised of activated T cells, as monitored by expression of the IL-2Rα chain and Ki67 (indicative of cycling cells), and expression of intracellular IL-2, IL-4 and IL-17. FOXP3+ T-Reg cells were also expanded.

Accordingly, if CTLA-4 is part of an IL-2-induced negative feedback loop that functions to restrict the production of IL-2 and other cytokines, then an induced deficiency in CTLA-4 gene expression should result in an increased and prolonged production of IL-2 and other cytokines, as observed. In addition, autoimmunity occurred in iKO mice, as monitored by detection of autoantibodies to insulin, gastric antigens and salivary antigens (RO52), thereby indicating a breakdown in self-nonself discrimination. In further experiments focused on autoimmunity, the loss of CTLA-4 in adulthood conferred enhanced susceptibility of collagen-induced arthritis, but paradoxically, protected mice from peptide-induced but not protein-induced allergic encephalomyelitis. A 2015, similar iKO study in a different mouse strain (C57BL/6), reported less severe lymphoproliferation, and also revealed increased expression of immune-inhibitory molecules, such as IL-10, LAG-3, and PD-1, providing potential compensatory inhibitory mechanisms attenuating the effects of the deleted CTLA-4 gene.[39] These experiments are particularly important, because they mirror the effects of the administration of CTLA-4 blocking MoAbs in human cancer immunotherapy: T cell-mediated systemic autoimmune "off target" side effects can be severe.

Systemic Autoimmunity: Loss of Negative Feedback Cytokine Control

Thus, after more than three decades of elucidation of the molecular mechanisms regulating immune responsiveness, it is now evident that regulation of the exquisite discriminative capacity of the immune system to recognize and react to nonself but not react to self lies predominantly at the level of negative feedback control of the reaction mediated by IL-2 and other cytokines, rather than the antigen recognition aspect of the system. It is to be especially noted that this represents a sea-change in thinking about how the immune reaction is regulated, and is contrary to Burnet's Clonal Selection Theory, which stressed the deletion of self-recognition lymphocyte clones as responsible for lack of self-reactivity.[40,41] Of course, cytokines were still yet to be described and discovered during Burnet's time. Also, this change in understanding of how the immune response is regulated has obvious therapeutic implications.

References

1. Miller J. (1961). Immunological function of the thymus. *Lancet* **2**:748–749.
2. Miller J. (1962). Effect of neonatal thymectomy on the immunological responsiveness of the mouse. *Proc Roy Soc London-B* **156**:415–428.
3. Sakaguchi S, Takahashi T and Nishizuka Y. (1982). Study on cellular events in post-thymectomy autoimmune oophoritis in mice. I. Requirement of Lyt-1 effector cells for oocytes damage after adoptive transfer. *J Exp Med* **156**:1565–1576.

4. Kisielow P, Hirst J, Shiku H, *et al.* (1975). Ly antigens as markers for functionally distinct subpopulations of thymus-derived lymphocytes of the mouse. *Nature* **253**:219–220.
5. Ledbetter J, Rouse R, Micklem H and Herzenberg L. (1980). T cell subsets defined by expression of Lyt1,2,3 and Thy1 antigens. Two parameter immunofluorescence and cytotoxicity analysis with monoclonal antibodies modifies current views. *J Exp Med* **152**:280.
6. Sakaguchi S, Takahashi T and Nishizuka Y. (1982). Study on cellular events in post-thymectomy autoimmune oophoritis in mice II. Requirement of Lyt-1 cells in normal female mice for prevention of oophoritis. *J Exp Med* **156**:1577–1586.
7. Sakaguchi S, Fukuma K, Kuribayashi K and Masuda T. (1985). Organ-specific autoimmune diseases induced in mice by elimination of T cell subset. I. Evidence for the active participation of T cells in natural self-tolerance; deficit of a T cell subset as a possible cause of autoimmune disease. *J Exp Med* **161**:72–87.
8. Schorle H, Holtschke T, Hunig T, *et al.* (1991). Development and function of T cells in mice rendered interleukin-2 deficient by gene targeting. *Nature* **352**:621–624.
9. Kundig TM, Schorle H, Bachmann MF, *et al.* (1993). Immune responses in interleukin-2-deficient mice. *Science* **262**:1059–1061.
10. Cousens LP, Orange JS, and Biron CA. (1995). Endogenous IL-2 contributes to T cell expansion and IFN-gamma production during lymphocytic choriomeningitis virus infection. *J Immunol* **155**:5690–5699.
11. Sadlack B, Lohler J, Schorle H, *et al.* (1995). Generalized autoimmune disease in interleukin-2-deficient mice is triggered by an uncontrolled activation and proliferation of CD4+ T cells. *Eur J Immunol* **25**: 3053–3059.
12. Horak I, Lohler J, Ma A, and Smith K. (1995). Interleukin-2 deficient mice: A new model to study autoimmunity and self-tolerance. *Immunol Rev* **148**:35–44.
13. Russell W, Russell L, and Gower J. (1959). Exceptional inheritance of a sex-linked gene in the mouse explained on the basis that the X/O sex-chromosome constitution is female. *PNAS* **45**:554–560.
14. Godfrey V, Wilkinson J and Russell L. (1991). X-linked lymphoreticular disease in the scurfy (sf) mutant mouse. *Am J Path* **138**:1379–1387.
15. Godfrey V, Rouse B and Wilkinson J. (1994). Transplantation of a T cell mediated lymphoreticular from the scurfy (sf) mouse disease. *Am J Path* **145**:281–286.

16. Blair P, Bultman S, Haas J, et al. (1994). CD4⁺CD8- T cells are the effector cells in disease pathogenesis in the scurfy (sf) mouse. *J Immunol* **153**:3764–3774.

17. Kanangat S, Blair P, Reddy R, et al. (1996). Disease in the scurfy (sf) mouse is associated with overexpression of cytokine genes. *E J Immunol* **26**:161–165.

18. Sakaguchi S, Sakaguchi N, Asano M, et al. (1995). Immunologic self-tolerance maintained by activated T cells expressing IL-2 receptor alpha-chains (CD25). Breakdown of a single mechanism of self-tolerance causes various autoimmune diseases. *J Immunol* **155**: 1151–1164.

19. Asano M, Toda M, Sakaguchi N and Sakaguchi S. (1996). Autoimmune disease as a consequence of developmental abnormality of a T cell sub-population. *J Exp Med* **184**:387–396.

20. Suri-Payer E, Amar A, Thornton A, and Shevach EM. (1998). CD4⁺CD25⁺ T cells inhibit both the induction and effector function of autoreactive T cells and represent a unique lineage of immunoregulatory T cells. *J Immunol* **160**:1212–1218.

21. Thornton AM and Shevach EM. (1998). CD4⁺CD25⁺ immunoregulatory T cells suppress polyclonal T cell activation *in vitro* by inhibiting inter-leukin 2 production. *J Exp Med* **188**:287–296.

22. Brunkow M, Jeffrey E, Hjerrild K, et al. (2001). Disruption of a new forkhead/winked-helix protein, scurfin, results in the fatal lymphoprolif-erative disorder of the scurfy mouse. *Nature Genet* **27**:68–73.

23. Chatlia T, Blaeser F, Ho N, et al. (2001). JM2, encoding a forkhead-related protein, is mutated in X-linked autoimmunity-allergic disregula-tion syndrome. *J Clin Invest* **106**:R75–R81.

24. Wildin R, Ramsdell F, Peake J, et al. (2001). X-linked neonatal diabe-tes mellitus, enteropathy and endocrinopathy syndrome is the human equivalent of mouse scurfy. *Nature Genet* **27**:18–20.

25. Bennet C, Christie J, Ramsdell M, et al. (2001). The immune dysregu-lation, polyendocrinopathy, enteropathy, X-linked syndrome (IPEX) is caused by mutations of FOXP3. *Nature Genet* **27**:20–21.

26. Schubert L, Jeffrey E, Zhang Y, et al. (2001). Scurfin (FOXP3) acts as a repressor of transcription and regulates T cell activation. *J Biol Chem* **276**:37672–37679.

27. Hori S, Nomura T and Sakaguchi S. (2003). Control of regulatory T cell development by the transcription factor FOXP3. *Science* **299**: 1057–1061.

28. Fontenot J, Gavin M and Rudensky A. (2003). FOXP3 programs the development and function of CD4$^+$CD25$^+$ regulatory T cells. *Nature Immunol* **4**:330–336.

29. Khattri R, Cox T, Yasayko S-A and Ramsdell F. (2003). An essential role for scurfin in CD4$^+$CD25$^+$ T regulatory cells. *Nature Immunol* **4**:337–342.

30. Smith K. (2010). *The Quantal Theory of Immunity: The Molecular Basis of Autoimmunity and Leukemia.* Singapore: World Scientific Publishing Co. Pte. Ltd. 243 pp.

31. Pandiyan P, Zheng L, Ishihara S, *et al.* (2007). CD4$^+$CD25$^+$FOXP3$^+$ regulatory T cells induce cytokine deprivation-mediated apoptosis of effector CD4$^+$ T cells. *Nat Immunol* **8**:1353–1362.

32. Feinerman O, Jentsch G, Sneddon M, *et al.* (2010). Single-cell quantification of IL-2 dynamics in effector and regulatory T cells reveals critical plasticity in immune responses. *Mol Sys Biol* **6**:437.

33. Smith KA and Cantrell DA. (1985). Interleukin 2 regulates its own receptors. *Proc Natl Acad Sci USA* **82**:864–868.

34. Nakajima H, Liu X-W, Wynshaw-Boris A, *et al.* (1997). An indirect effect of Stat5a in IL2-induced proliferation: A critical role for Stat5a in IL2-mediated IL2 receptor alpha chain induction. *Immunity* **7**:691–701.

35. Alegre M, Noel P, Eisfelder B, *et al.* (1996). Regulation of surface and intracellular expression of CTLA4 on mouse T cells. *J Immunol* **157**:4762–4770.

36. Hwang KW, Sweatt WB, Mashayekhi M, *et al.* (2004). Transgenic expression of CTLA-4 controls lymphoproliferation in IL-2-deficient mice. *J Immunol* **173**:5415–5424.

37. Wing K, Onishi Y, Preito-Martin P, *et al.* (2008). CTLA-4 control over FOXP3$^+$ regulatory cell function. *Science* **322**:271–275.

38. Klocke K, Sakaguchi S, Holmdahl R, and Wing K. (2016). Induction of autoimmune disease by deletion of CTLA-4 in mice in adulthood. *Proc Natl Acad Sci USA* **113**:E2382–2392.

39. Paterson A, Lovitch S, Sage P, *et al.* (2015). Deletion of CTLA-4 on regulatory T cells during adulthood leads to resistance to autoimmunity. *J Exp Med* 1–19.

40. Burnet FM. (1957). A modification of Jerne's theory of antibody production using the concept of clonal selection. *Aust J Sci* **20**:67–77.

41. Burnet FM. (1959). *The Clonal Selection Theory of Acquired Immunity.* Cambridge: Cambridge University Press.

9 Immunotherapy

Coley's Toxins and "Active Immunotherapy"

The dream of harnessing the immune system to attack cancers originated more than a century ago in 1893 when William Coley reported about his experience injecting cancer patients with live bacteria and heat-killed bacterial extracts.[1] This idea was based on his observations of some of his cancer patients who became infected with TB or other serious bacterial infections and that subsequently appeared to undergo complete remissions from their tumors. Although all injected patients developed high fevers, and some experienced septic shock, a small fraction, on the order of 5%–10%, had subsequent complete disappearance of all tumors, and many of these individuals were apparently cured with no relapses over long time intervals. At the time, Coley took some of his patients to medical meetings to show his fellow physicians that his treatments resulted in complete tumor disappearance. Many of his colleagues tried his therapy, which came to be known as "Coley's Toxins." However, the toxic reactions suffered by the subjects precluded widespread adoption of the procedure.

Subsequently, in 1902 Paul Portier and Charles Richet discovered allergic reactions to the prophylactic repetitive injections of toxins, some of which led to death due to anaphylactic shock.[2] Also, in 1908 Clemmons von Pirquet and Bela Shick published a monumental work describing "serum sickness," resulting from injections of hyper-immune horse serum raised against diphtheria and streptococcal organisms in efforts to use "serotherapy" for these lethal infections.[3] Moreover, with the advent of radiotherapy in the early decades of the 20th century, a new modality was introduced that was much less toxic, and resulted in shrinkage of tumors in almost all patients, although few if any cures resulted. Even so, immunology became a science relegated to more fundamental approaches to understand how the immune system functions and dreams of the early immunotherapists to eradicate both cancers and infectious diseases were never realized.

Half a century passed before a report by Georges Mathe and his colleagues introduced the concept of "active immunotherapy" of cancer in 1969, describing the use of the bovine TB vaccine Bacillus Calmette Guerin (BCG),[4] combined with injections of irradiated allogeneic leukemia cells in acute lymphoblastic leukemia (ALL) patients.[5] The rationale of this active immunotherapy was drawn from the use bacterial Coley's Toxins to "nonspecifically augment" immune reactions using the bacteria, and simultaneously to expose the host immune system to putative tumor-specific antigens (TSAs) derived from the allogeneic leukemic blast cells. These tumor-specific antigens were assumed to exist based upon animal leukemias and sarcomas induced by RNA tumor viruses, which shared viral antigens.[6] Care was taken to first reduce the tumor burden with chemotherapy as much as possible before immunotherapy was introduced. This single report ushered in an era of enthusiasm for cancer immunotherapy that has persisted to the present time. Unfortunately, repeat large scale trials of BCG + allogeneic leukemia cell active immunotherapy a la Mathe failed to show the efficacy reported in the initial trials. It was never clear why the subsequent trials failed to show an antitumor effect, or whether the BCG or the allogeneic leukemic cells was the most important component of the therapy. Mathe maintained that his detractors failed to use the proper strain of BCG that he had obtained from the Pasteur Institute.

Cytotoxic T Lymphocyte Lines and Clones-Adoptive Immunotherapy

Almost ten years later in 1977, we reported that it as possible to generate tumor-specific CTL by a combination of *in vivo* immunization of mice with allogeneic RNA tumor virus transformed leukemic cells, followed by *in vitro* repetitive short-term allogeneic mixed tumor lymphocyte cultures (MTLC).[7] Of importance, the CTLs generated were found to not only lyse allogeneic tumors induced by Friend Leukemia Virus (FLV), but also syngeneic FLV leukemia cells. Thus, following Mathe's lead, one could use the strong MHC-encoded alloantigens to augment recognition of the presumptive weaker tumor/virus-specific antigens. Then, we found that we could maintain such tumor-specific CTL in continuous culture, apparently indefinitely, by seeding the activated cells into medium containing T Cell Growth Factor (TCGF),[8] thereby creating Cytotoxic T Lymphocyte Lines (CTLL)[9] and clones.[10] This advance opened the way to a new approach to immunotherapy, allowing an extension of Mathe's "active immunotherapy" to "adoptive immunotherapy," as described originally by Billingham in 1962.[11] Accordingly, after the *in vivo/in vitro* selection of CTLL, and their TCGF expansion *in vitro*, their adoptive transfer to tumor bearing hosts became feasible for the first time.

Even though theoretically feasible, the practicality of growing large numbers of tumor-specific CTLL *in vitro* necessitated a reproducible source of the TCGF. Accordingly, armed with the quantitative TCGF bioassay that we reported in 1978,[8] we purified enough active molecules[12] to immunize mice and produced TCGF-reactive MoAbs that we then used to immunoaffinity purify milligram quantities of homogeneous molecules that were termed interleukin-2 (IL-2) molecules for the first time in 1983.[13] Also, we radiolabeled purified IL-2 molecules, which enabled the creation of a radiolabeled-IL-2 binding assay reported in 1981 and the characterization of IL-2 receptors, which were detectable only on antigen-activated T cells.[14] Then, the IL-2 molecular characteristics (MW 15.5 kDa, pI 8.2) and the IL-2 bioassay permitted the identification of a cDNA encoding a molecule with the appropriate molecular characteristics and activity in 1983.[15]

High Dose IL-2 Immunotherapy

The approaches to immunotherapy initiated by Coley and Mathe assumed that tumors express tumor specific antigens, but that these antigens were relatively weak immunogens, thereby necessitating adjuvants such as bacterial extracts/BCG to nonspecifically augment immune recognition and reactivity. Steven Rosenberg added further to this rationale, taking advantage of the availability of recombinant IL-2 (rIL-2) for use as a non-antigen specific adjuvant to boost immunoreactivity. In 1985, Rosenberg's group reported their experience with the administration of huge rIL-2 doses (~2 mg IV) every 8 hours (so-called "high dose IL-2 therapy") to 25 subjects with various metastatic cancers (7-melanoma, 9-colorectal, 4-sarcomas, 3-renal, 1-lung adenocarcinoma, 1-esophageal) together with the administration of autologous PBMCs cultured in IL-2 for 3-4 days.[16] These cells were termed Lymphokine-Activated Killer (LAK) cells, because they could be shown to lyse both Natural Killer cell (NK-cell) tumor targets as well as non-NK cell tumor targets *in vitro,* and they lacked markers for both T cells and B cells. Rosenberg aspired to the generation of tumor antigen-specific CTL, but he had no way to select for T cells reactive with putative tumor antigen specificities, so that he defaulted to simply culturing PBMCs in IL-2 for 3–4 days and terming them LAK cells. It is noteworthy that LAK cells were never given a recognizable phenotype so that their origin and function remained obscure. However, because IL-2 was used to generate their killer activity, presumably some LAK cells expressed IL-2Rs.

Eleven of the 25 subjects were reported to have measurable tumor regression (at least 50% decrease of tumor volume), but all subjects needed circulatory support due to hypotension, so that 80% of the subjects gained >10% of their body weight due to fluid retention, accompanied by pulmonary edema, hypoxemia and dyspnea. These severe side effects, accompanied by fever, chills and generalized malaise, were recognizable as the systemic inflammatory response syndrome, or septic shock, like the symptoms experienced by subjects treated with Coley's Toxins. Rosenberg attributed the toxicities due to the IL-2 treatment rather than the LAK cells based upon other data of the administration of IL-2 alone and LAK cells alone.[16] We now know that these shock symptoms result from the high doses of IL-2 administered, which result in high systemic IL-2 concentrations that saturate both IL-2 and IL-15 receptors (IL-15R) expressed by NK cells[17] as well as memory CD8+ T cells,[18] and which then release large quantities of pro-inflammatory cytokines, such as INFγ, IL-6 and TNFα. Accordingly, high concentrations of circulating pro-inflammatory cytokines are responsible for the circulatory collapse of septic shock, whether initiated by bacteremia, LPS, Coley's Toxins or high dose IL-2. The question therefore becomes the mechanism(s) responsible for tumor regressions seen. In this regard, Rosenberg stated repeatedly that "the toxicity IS the therapy."

Two years later in 1987, now 30 years ago at the time of this writing, Rosenberg summarized their experience with adoptive immunotherapy using LAK cells and IL-2 vs. high dose IL-2 alone in the treatment of 157 subjects with advanced cancer.[19] Of 106 subjects who received the combination therapy, an objective response (>50% decrease in all lesions) was observed in 22%, including 8 subjects in whom all cancer regressed completely. Of those 45 subjects who received high dose IL-2 (~2 mg q8h IV) alone, there were 6 objective responses (13%), including one complete response. As in the initial report, these subjects all experienced the severe side effects of high dose IL-2 therapy. In this regard, these results, both in terms of a tumor response, as well as the universal toxicity, are quite similar to those reported by Coley almost a century earlier.[1] Also, from these results, it is noteworthy that the high dose IL-2 therapy alone yielded anti-tumor responses. Whether the LAK cells added to the response rate required additional studies and subjects.

A decade earlier in 1977, Eva Klein and colleagues had reported that most tumor infiltrating lymphocytes (TIL) in humans are immunologically nonreactive, despite reactivity in the peripheral blood lymphocytes (PBL).[20] Subsequently, in 1985 E. Carmack Holmes reported on whether circulating PBL reflected accurately the phenotype and immunological reactivity of TILs from human pulmonary tumors.[21] As far as their surface markers were concerned, the percentage of T cells, B cells, Th cells, CTL and NK cells were found to be similar in the two compartments. However, the TIL were markedly suppressed in their functional capacity, as measured by their proliferative and cytotoxic activity. Particularly noteworthy, NK cell activity was markedly diminished in TIL compared with PBL. A similar lack of reactivity of TIL was reported by von Fleidner and co-workers in studies of 22 humans with solid tumors in 1986.[22] These investigators conjectured "that tumor cells may inhibit certain functions of the TIL in human solid tumors."

By comparison, Rosenberg's team reported in 1988 that TIL expanded in IL-2 and adoptively transferred to mice bearing metastases from various types of tumors were 50–100 times more effective in their therapeutic potency than LAK cells.[23] Based on these data, Rosenberg and co-workers ignored the earlier work by others regarding TIL, and reported in 1986 on 20 subjects with metastatic melanoma treated with a single dose of Cytoxan, followed in 36 hours by the infusion of 2×10^{11} TIL that had been cultured with IL-2, and then administered IV IL-2 (10^5 U/Kg body weight = 7×10^6 U $\cong$ 2 mg) every 8 hours for 5 days.[24] Regression of cancer was observed in 11/20 subjects (55%), however, these regressions were transient, lasting from 2–13 months.

Rosenberg's group also continued to treat subjects with metastatic cancer with high dose IV IL-2 therapy with and without LAK cells. Their experience in 652 cancer patients was reported in 1989.[25] Their results confirmed those reported previously: of 130 evaluable subjects who received IL-2 alone, there were 4 CR (3%) and 18 PR (14%), while of 177 evaluable subjects who received IL-2+ LAK cells, there were 14 CR (8%) and 30 PR (17%). Toxicity in these subjects, like those reported earlier was severe, with 508 of 652 (78%) requiring vasopressors for hypotension. There were 22 episodes of angina, 6 myocardial infarcts, 78 arrythmias, and 10 deaths because of the therapy. From these results, it could be concluded that IL-2 alone was certainly effective in a small fraction of subjects, but it remained unclear as to whether the LAK cell infusions added any efficacy.

Accordingly, the Rosenberg group launched a prospective, randomized controlled trial comparing high dose IL-2 therapy alone vs. IL-2 in conjunction with LAK cells that they reported in 1993.[26] There were 97 subjects with metastatic renal cell cancer, and 54 subjects had metastatic malignant melanoma for a total of 181 subjects entered on trial. Like the previous report, there were not significant differences comparing the two therapies: of evaluable subjects, IL-2 therapy alone (79 subjects) yielded 4 CRs and 12 PRs, while IL-2+

LAK (85 subjects) yielded 10 CRs and 14 PRs. Consequently, LAK cells were omitted from future trials, and the Rosenberg group's attention was turned to TILs in hopes to improve the frequencies of responses that could be achieved with IL-2 alone.

Adoptive Cell Therapy (ACT)-Chimeric Antigen Receptor (CAR) T Cells

Although our 1977 report of the generation and long-term growth of tumor-specific CTL[9] and their subsequent clonal isolation reported in 1979[10] provided the means for adoptive cell therapy (ACT) that we speculated might be used to treat humans with cancer, the lack of defined tumor-specific antigens (TSAs) expressed by human cancer cells was a major obstacle. In our murine experiments, we took advantage of using allogeneic Friend Leukemia Virus (FLV)-induced leukemia cells as immunogens of normal mice to augment immune responses to FLV-specified antigens, which were also expressed by syngeneic leukemia cells.[7,27] Almost two decades later, in 1995, Cliona Rooney and co-workers reported that it was possible to generate Epstein Barr Virus (EBV)-specific CTL lines from allogeneic donors of bone marrow transplants (BMT) that could be used successfully to treat BMT recipients with EBV-related lymphoproliferative disease.[27] EBV-specific CTL were generated from donor PBMCs activated *in vitro* with EBV-transformed B-lymphoblastoid cell lines, then expanded by culturing with IL-2. Of 10 subjects treated, one individual with an EBV+ immunoblastic lymphoma had a complete resolution of disease after four CTL infusions (two $1 \times 10^7/m^2$ and two $5 \times 10^7/m^2$). Accordingly, this report, and an additional report of the successful treatment of cytomegalovirus (CMV) in BMT recipients,[28] showed that ACT using virus-specific lines and clones of CD8+ CTL is a safe and effective way to reconstitute cellular immunity against viruses and virus-induced tumors after allogeneic bone marrow transplantation.

Although these reports showed the feasibility of ACT for viral infections, a remaining major impediment to cancer immunotherapy was the lack of identified human tumor-specific or tumor-associated antigens. As an initial approach to this problem, in 1993 Zelig Eshar and co-workers sought to circumvent this hurdle by creating Chimeric Antigen Receptors (CAR) in T cells.[29] The rationale was based on using a single chain variable region fragment (scFv) of a MoAb. To activate T cells, genes encoding this antibody-antigen-binding domain were linked to the gene segments encoding the CD3ζ chain, which could transmit the TCR activating signal. Because many MoAbs were already available, the idea was to endow T cells with antibody-type recognition. As a model system, they used chimeric genes for an anti-2,4,6-trinitrophenyl (TNP) scFv and the CD3ζ chain. CTL hybridomas expressing such chimeric scFv-ζ genes interacted specifically with TNP-modified target cells, underwent activation as monitored by IL-2 production, and subsequently killed specifically TNP-modified target cells.

Two years later, in 1995 Bejcek and co-workers reported the construction of recombinant single chain antibody fragments (scFvs) directed against CD19,[30] which is known to be expressed by all normal B cells, but also by most B cell malignancies, including acute lymphoblastic leukemia (ALL), chronic lymphocytic leukemia (CLL) and most B cell lymphomas. Thus, CD19 could be thought of as a tumor-associated antigen (TAA), which if it could be targeted with CAR T cells, would generate a new ACT for B cell leukemias and lymphomas. Accordingly, in 2003 Michel Sadelain's group constructed a CD19-CD3-ζ-specific CAR and sub-cloned it into a retroviral (gibbon ape LV) vector, which they used to infect mitogen-activated human PBLs.[31] These cells were selected on APCs transduced to express CD19 and CD80, the B7 ligand for the co-stimulatory molecule CD28. After expansion with IL-15, these CAR T cells persisted in human tumor-bearing SKID-Beige mice, which lack T cells, B cells and NK cells, and eradicated disseminated intramedullary tumors. Accordingly, the tools for ACT of human B cell malignancies were at hand.

Subsequently, in 2006 Claudia Kowolick improved upon this CAR T cell construct by a 2nd generation CD19 CAR, which included a modified chimeric CD28 signaling domain fused to chimeric CD3-ζ. The CD19RCD28⁺ T cells specifically lysed CD19⁺ tumor cells *in vitro*, and after stimulation by CD19⁺ tumor cells, produced

IL-2 and proliferated without exogenous IL-2 supplementation, and, after adoptive transfer to tumor-bearing mice, these CD19RCD28+ T cells showed an improved persistence and anti-tumor effect compared with CD19R+ T cells.

By 2010, there were clinical trials at seven sites in the U.S. in which subjects were given infusions of T cells modified to express CARs against the CD19 molecule present on most B-lineage leukemias and lymphomas.[32] A workshop with all of the principal groups attending was held in Bethesda, MD to summarize the progress and problems associated with CAR T cell therapy.[32] A total of 18 treated subjects were tallied as of May 2010, and excellent clinical responses were reported anecdotally in several of the trials, even though most of the subjects entered on trial were end-stage patients, having failed all standard therapies. However, one serious adverse event (SAEs) had already occurred in a CLL patient. The SAE consisted of a cytokine storm syndrome, with acute sepsis, renal failure and resultant shock, and accompanied by acute respiratory distress syndrome. It was noted that although CD19 is only expressed on normal B cells, the investigators felt that although CD19 CAR T cells may inadvertently eliminate a patient's normal B cells, this side effect could be ameliorated with IV gamma globulin replacement.

Fast forward to 2017, at least three companies started CD19-CAR T cell programs (Juno, Kite and Novartis). In clinical trials Juno had three deaths in a trial for ALL, and subsequently discontinued it, while their efforts continue in lymphoma. The deaths were due to cerebral edema, which has been traced to a predominant cerebral cytokine release syndrome.[33] Pro-inflammatory CSF cytokine concentrations have been found as much as 20-200-fold higher than those in peripheral blood. By comparison, Novartis recently received a positive evaluation by the FDA Oncologic Drugs Advisory Committee for the use of CD19-CAR T cells for the treatment of ALL. Overall, CD19-CAR T cell therapy in B cell malignancies is effective, notwithstanding difficulties inherent in the introduction of any new treatment modality.

The initial CD19 scFvs used were derived from murine MoAbs, so that difficulties arose because of human immune responses to the murine-specified proteins, both humoral as well as T cell mediated, which truncated the survival of the CD19 CAR T cells, and thereby led to malignant relapses. Accordingly, efforts are now directed to developing human CD19 scFvs.[34] Another complication is malignant relapse because of mutational escape from the epitope recognized by the anti-CD19 scFv. Like antimicrobial therapy and chemotherapy, present day immunotherapists have come to appreciate the power of immunological polyclonal epitope recognition, both humoral and cellular-mediated. Future immunotherapies may well evolve into combinatorial epitope recognition clones of CAR T cells. An additional complication is the systemic cytokine release syndrome, thought to be due to CD19 CAR T cell activation by both a high tumor burden and significant expression of CD19 on normal B cells. Moreover, immunodeficiency due to the loss of normal B cells, even though compensated by the administration of IV Ig, may prove to be a significant problem as time goes on. The use of tumor associated antigens instead of tumor-specific antigens (which remain elusive) may prove difficult for other tumor associated antigens, such as HER-2 which is also expressed by normal lung cells. B cells may be expendable, but lung cells, not so much. Thus, whether CAR T cells will prove to be the major break-through hoped for, time will tell.

Adoptive Cell Therapy-TCR Gene Transfer

It is clear from the observed efficacy of CD19 CAR T cell ACT that T cells can be very effective against tumors, even established and metastatic malignancies. However, as discussed above, the difficulty remains in identifying tumor-specific antigens to target, either with Ab-derived antigen recognition reagents or, more physiologically, via TCRs. Paul Allen and co-workers reported in 2000 a murine model system utilizing a methylcholanthrene–induced fibrosarcoma.[35] This chemically-induced tumor had a previously identified nonamer peptide derived from a mutated ERK2 kinase.[36] Allen's group generated TCR transgenic mice with TCR reactivity to this mutated peptide and tested these T cells in ACT. They found that eradication of established tumors by adoptive transfer of the TCR transgenic T cells was possible, but it was T cell/tumor cell dose and time-dependent. Thus, given a known tumor-specific antigen and known tumor-specific antigen-reactive CD8+ T cells, ACT works.

Subsequently, in 2001 Ton Schumacher and co-workers used a model murine system to test the notion that TCR gene transfer could be used to redirect the T cell antigen specificity to be used for ACT.[37] They selected TCR α and β genes that encoded a TCR that recognized an epitope from the nucleoprotein of influenza virus, which were inserted into a MLV retroviral vector and used to infect splenocytes *in vitro*. After the short-term *in vitro* culture, 5-15% of total CD8+ T cells expressed the introduced TCR as tested by tetramer staining via flow cytometry. These cell populations were injected IV (1.8×10^7) of which ~9% were tetramer+ (2.7×10^5), and then two days later mice were challenged by the injection of the appropriate strain of Flu virus and control strains. A marked expansion of tetramer+ cells occurred only in mice that received virus with the immunogenic nucleoprotein. To test whether ACT could be directed towards tumor cells, EL4 lymphoma cells that expressed the Flu epitope were treated with tetramer+ T cells (only 28×10^3), which rapidly eradicated previously inoculated tumor cells. Accordingly, based on these and additional data, Schumacher concluded that *"the redirection of T cells by TCR gene transfer is a viable strategy for the rapid induction of virus- or tumor-specific immunity."*

Despite these proof of concept results, the identification of TSAs expressed on the surface of human tumors that could be used to create tumor-specific T cells by TCR gene transfer has remained problematic. Rosenberg's group expended a lot of effort in culturing TILs from metastatic melanomas in hopes to identify tumor-specific antigens. However, in 2009 they reported that the CD8+ TILs found in melanomas express high levels of the co-inhibitory molecule PD-1 and in addition, these cells are functionally impaired,[38] as one would expect from "exhausted T cells" exposed to persistent antigens.[39] Accordingly, by 2015, there were 34 biotech/pharma companies involved in ACT projects, but only three of them had projects on TCR gene transfer that reacted with tumor-associated antigens (cancer testes antigen NY-ESO-1, WT-1, "autologous antigen"), the remainder all focused on CD19-reactive CARs.[40] Tumor-specific antigens have remained elusive.

Checkpoint Inhibitors-Anti-CTLA-4

As already detailed, the discovery of T cell co-inhibitory receptor molecules such as CTLA-4 and PD-1, as well as the initial murine experiments demonstrating the anti-tumor efficacy of MoAbs blocking these inhibitory receptors in murine tumor model systems, the rationale for testing these so-called "checkpoint inhibitors" in human cancer became inevitable. Thus, a human MoAb capable of blocking CTLA-4 binding to its ligand (B7) was developed by Thomas Davis, and administered to subjects with metastatic melanoma by Rosenberg's team, with the first results reported in 2003.[41] Every three weeks, subjects received anti-CTLA-4 MoAb at 3 mg/kg IV over 90 minutes, followed by a vaccine, consisting of 1 mg each of two peptides derived from a melanoma-associated antigen (gp100) emulsified in incomplete Freund's adjuvant and administered subcutaneously. It was intended to enroll 21 subjects, but accrual was terminated after 14 subjects were entered, because of the development of grade III/IV autoimmune toxicity: six of 14 subjects (43%) developed grade III/IV autoimmune toxicities, including severe dermatitis (3 subjects), colitis/enterocolitis (2 subjects) and one subject each with hypophysitis and hepatitis. Accordingly, these toxicities were entirely different from the cytokine storms seen after Coley's Toxins, high dose IL-2 administration, or CD19 CAR infusions, and led to the conclusion that the results *"establish a clear role for CTLA-4 in the maintenance of peripheral tolerance in humans."* Of course, these results were predictable, given the 1995 reports of severe systemic autoimmunity occurring in CTLA-4 (-/-) mice.[42,43] Also, the autoimmune syndromes suffered by the subjects with melanoma who received CTLA-4 blocking MoAbs as adults were subsequently recapitulated in the inducible CTLA-4 gene deletion of adult mice in 2016.[44]

However, two of the first melanoma subjects who received CTLA-4 blocking MoAb experienced complete tumor responses, while one subject had a partial response.[41] Thus, in addition to suppressing immune recognition and responses to self-antigens, the results from the first CTLA-4 blocking trial revealed that doing so would lead to anti-tumor immune responses. Despite the reported toxicities, blocking anti-CTLA-4 administration clearly led to anti-tumor activity, and held the promise of long-term responses.

Accordingly, a randomized, double blind, phase-3 trial of anti-CTLA-4 in subjects with metastatic melanoma was conducted in 125 centers in 13 countries between 2004 and 2008 and published in 2010.[45] The subjects were randomly assigned, in a 3:1:1 ratio to receive anti-CTLA-4 + gp100 (403 subjects), anti-CTLA-4 alone (137 subjects), or gp100 alone (136 subjects). The MoAb was administered at a dose of 3 mg/kg and subjects received the MoAb+/- gp100 every 3 weeks for a total of four treatments. The primary endpoint of this trial was survival. The median overall survival was ~10 months for the groups that received anti-CTLA-4 vs. 6.4 months for the group that received only gp100 ($P < 0.001$). It was concluded that anti-CTLA-4 therapy improved survival in patients with metastatic melanoma, leading to approval by the U.S. Food and Drug Administration (FDA) in 2011.

However, for a few more months survival, ~60% of the subjects who received the MoAb experienced immune-related adverse events (AEs) with 10–15% suffering grade 3–4 events, i.e. serious adverse events (SAEs). The most common AEs affected the skin and GI tract. Most of the SAEs were attributed to extreme rashes with pruritus, colitis requiring corticosteroid anti-inflammatory/immunosuppressive therapy, and hypophysitis requiring hormone replacement therapy. Also, in many subjects who survived beyond 2-years and had suffered SAEs during the administration phase, the symptoms persisted. In 2013, a retrospective study of 752 subjects who had received anti-CTLA-4 therapy identified a total of 120 AEs (16%), which were classified according to organ system.[46] Skin reactions were common, with many subjects suffering from maculopapular rashes. Rarely, Sweet's syndrome, Stevens-Johnson syndrome/toxic epidermal lysis was observed. Diarrhea due to colitis is a common AE. Severe colitis can result in bowel perforation or intractable bleeding requiring colectomy. Hepatotoxicity is reported in 3–9% of treated patients and usually manifests as an asymptomatic increase of transaminases and bilirubin. However, hepatitis can be severe with fatal liver failure, so that grade 3–4 hepatotoxicity had to be treated with glucocorticoids. As to the endocrine system, thyroiditis is common, presenting as either hypo or hyperthyroidism. Also, hypophysitis is not a common AE but can be quite severe. Neurological dysfunction is rare, but can be very serious. Common symptoms include headache, dizziness, lethargy, and asthenia. Rarely, patients can present with cranial neuropathy, optic nerve ischemia, ataxia, tremor, myoclonia, dysarthria, and peripheral neuropathy. Guillian-Barre syndrome is infrequent but can be fatal. Respiratory tract AEs can include severe pneumonitis, fatal acute respiratory distress syndrome (ARDS), pulmonary granulomatosis, and sarcoidosis.

Thus, the question of efficacy regarding anti-CTLA-4 therapy for metastatic melanoma evolved from one of prolonged survival of those receiving immunotherapy to the potential long-term disease-free interval for a subset of subjects. Historically, the median overall survival (OS) was 8–10 months with conventional chemotherapy, so that the median OS for anti-CTLA-4 therapy is not that much different compared to historical data. Therefore, to gain a more accurate estimate of the benefit of therapy, Dirk Schadendorf and colleagues performed a pooled analysis of OS data in 2015 for 1,861 subjects from 12 studies: the median OS was 11.4 months, and the Kaplan-Meier OS curve revealed a plateau beginning around year 3, when the survival rate was 21%, which extended up to 10 years in some subjects.[47] Considering the historical 5-year survival of ~10%, these data revealed a potential for a doubling of the frequency of long-term survivors with metastatic melanoma, but no substantial benefit for the remainder 80% of patients. As pointed out by the authors, these data were derived from multiple studies, conducted in different eras, spanning a period of ~10 years. Also, as noted, these data are OS data, so that it is unknown whether the long-term survivors were indeed tumor-free and thus "cured." Also, just as in subjects who are long-term survivors of high dose IL-2 therapy, the characteristics that differentiate the responders vs. the non-responders remained unknown.

Checkpoint Inhibitors-Anti-PD-1/PDL-1

In 2012, two reports detailed the results of phase I dose-finding trials testing MoAbs reactive to the co-inhibitory lymphocyte receptor Programmed Death one (PD-1) and to the ligand PDL-1 in subjects with advanced cancer. The first report from Suzanne Topalian and others,[48] dealt with anti-PD-1 MoAb administered at 0.01–10.0 mg/kg every two weeks. Response was assessed after each 8-week treatment cycle. Subjects received as many as 12 cycles until disease progression or a complete response occurred. A total of 296 subjects received treatment, and among 236 subjects in whom response could be evaluated, objective responses (CR or PR) occurred (all doses) in 18% of non-small cell lung cancer, 28% of melanoma, and 27% of renal cell cancer. There were no responses in prostate or colorectal cancer. Many responses appeared durable: 20 of 31 responses lasted >1 year in subjects with >1 year of follow-up.

Regarding toxicity, there were no signs or symptoms indicative of cytokine storm as occurs in high dose IL-2 or anti-CD19 CAR therapy. Grade 3 or 4 treatment-related AEs were observed in 41 of 296 subjects (14%). The drug-related SAEs, which occurred in 32 of 296 subjects (11%), and were deemed of probable immune-related causes, included inflammatory pneumonitis, vitiligo, colitis, hepatitis, hypophysitis, and thyroiditis, and thus similar to those SAEs seen with anti-CTLA-4 therapy. Noteworthy was the finding that immunohistochemical analysis of pre-treatment tumor specimens, of 17 subjects with PD-L1-negative tumors, none had objective responses, while 9 of 25 subjects with PD-L1-positive tumors, had an objective response.

Julie Brahmer and colleagues reported their experience with a multicenter phase 1 study of a PDL-1-blocking human MoAb.[49] The MoAb was administered to 207 subjects at escalating doses ranging from 0.3–10 mg/kg every 14 days for up to 16 cycles or until a complete response or disease progression occurred. Among subjects with a response that could be evaluated, an objective response (CR or PR) occurred in 9/52 (17%) of subjects with melanoma, 2/17 (12%) subjects with renal cell cancer, 5/49 (10%) subjects with non-small cell lung cancer, and 1/17 (6%) subjects with ovarian cancer. Responses lasted for >1 year in 8/16 subjects with at least 1 year of follow-up. Drug-related AEs occurred in 39% of subjects and included rash, hypothyroidism, hepatitis, sarcoidosis, endophthalmitis, diabetes mellitus and myasthenia gravis. Treatment-related SAEs occurred in only 5% of subjects. None of the subjects suffered from cytokine storm. Accordingly, the immune-related AEs were less frequent, milder and qualitatively different from those observed with anti-CTLA-4 therapy, consistent with reports of gene deletion experiments in mice. For example, severe colitis, an SAE seen in anti-CTLA-4 and anti-PD-1 therapies was infrequent in subjects receiving anti-PDL-1.

In 2015, Caroline Robert and colleagues reported their experience with a randomized, controlled multicenter phase 3 study, comparing two doses of blocking PD-1 MoAb (10 mg/kg every two or three weeks) with anti-CTLA-4 (3 mg/kg every 3 weeks) in advanced melanoma. Primary endpoints were progression-free and overall survival. There was no significant difference between the two PD-1 MoAb regimens, and both were superior to the CTLA-4 MoAb: response rates were 33.7% for PD-1 MoAb every two weeks and 32.9% every 3 weeks vs. 11.9% for the anti-CTLA-4 MoAb. Rates of CRs were 5%, 6.1% and 1.4%. Treatment-related SAEs were lower in the anti-PD-1groups (13.3% and 10.1%) than in the anti-CTLA-4 group (19.9%). Thus, blocking the PD-1/PDL-1 pathway is superior to blocking CTLA-4 in melanoma, but the responses occur in only a subset of individuals.

Also in 2015, Larkin and colleagues reported a randomized double-blind, phase 3 study in 945 advanced melanoma subjects, comparing anti-PD-1 alone vs. combined anti-PD-1 + anti-CTLA-4 vs. anti-CTLA-4 alone.[50] Progression-free survival and overall survival were co-primary endpoints. Only the progression-free survivals were reported. The median progression-free survival with the combination = 11.5 months vs. 6.9 months for anti-PD-1 alone vs. 2.9 months for anti-CTLA-4 alone. Treatment related SAEs occurred in 16.3% of subjects in the anti-PD-1 alone group vs. 55.0% in the combination group vs. 27.3% in the anti-CTLA-4 alone group, diarrhea/colitis being the most frequent SAE.

The higher frequency of SAEs in the group that received combined anti-CTLA-4 and anti-PD-1 MoAbs may well preclude this approach to try to improve outcomes. A recent report of two individuals who suffered fulminant myocarditis from the combination[51] recalls the earlier observations of CTLA-4 (-/-) mice that developed a T cell-mediated myocarditis, and PD-1 (-/-) mice that developed an antibody-mediated myocarditis. Both the individuals reported had extensive T cell (both CD4[+] and CD8[+]) infiltration of the myocardium and skeletal muscle, thus indicative of T cell-mediated inflammation rather than humoral damage.

As in high dose IL-2 therapy, only a subset of individuals responded to checkpoint inhibitor therapy, and it was not clear how these individuals could be differentiated from those who did not respond. Thus, a 2015 report from Naiyer Rizvi and colleagues regarding the frequency of mutations in determining sensitivity to PD-1 blockade in non-small cell lung cancer (NSCLC) was especially important.[52] They used whole exome sequencing of two independent cohorts of NSCLC and found that higher nonsynonymous mutation burden in tumors was associated with improved objective response, durable clinical benefit, and progression-free survival. Efficacy also correlated with the molecular smoking signature, higher neoantigen burden and DNA repair pathway mutations. Thus, the greater the frequency of mutations, the greater likelihood that immune checkpoint inhibitors may offer benefit. However, if the tumor does not express neo-antigens bound to MHC-encoded HLA molecules on the cell surface, lowering the threshold for TCR activation will not lead to a tumor-specific T cell-mediated immune response.

Subsequently, in 2017 Dung Le and colleagues evaluated the efficacy of PD-1 blockade in subjects with advanced mismatch repair (MMR)-deficient cancers across 12 different tumor types.[53] Eighty-six consecutive subjects were enrolled between September 2013 and September 2016. Objective radiographic responses were noted in 53% of subjects, with 21% achieving a complete radiographic response. The average time to any response was 21 weeks and the average time to complete response was 42 weeks. They also directly tested the hypothesis that checkpoint blockade induces peripheral expansion of tumor-specific T cells and that MMR-deficient tumors harbor functional mutation-associated neo-antigens. Deep sequencing of CDR3 regions (TCRseq) was performed on tumors from three responding subjects. Intra-tumoral T cell clones were found that were selectively expanded in the periphery after treatment initiation. They estimated the fraction of cancer patients that might benefit from this kind of approach, and found that >5% of adenocarcinomas of the endometrium, stomach, small intestine, colon and rectum, cervix, prostate, bile duct and liver, neuroendocrine tumors, non-epithelial ovarian cancers, and uterine sarcomas were MMR-deficient. This represents roughly 40,000 stage I-III and 20,000 stage IV diagnoses in the U.S.

If co-inhibitory receptors such as CTLA-4 and PD-1 normally function via the suppression of TCR signal transduction, dampening production of IL-2 and other cytokines, it is not clear why immune checkpoint blockade does not lead to a cytokine storm such as occurs during high dose IL-2 administration and CD19 CAR T cell administration. The explanation may reside in the kinetics of the anti-tumor response to checkpoint blockade, which evolves over several months via the expansion of tumor-specific T cells, rather than occurring immediately upon the IV introduction of IL-2, or CD19 CAR T cells.

Therapeutic Tumor-Specific Vaccines

The quintessence of the problem of tumor immunology remains the question of whether the tumor cells express neoantigens that can be recognized as foreign by the immune system. If not, then boosting immune/inflammatory responses nonspecifically will result in nothing more than toxicity, without a therapeutic response. Accordingly, the holy grail is to create a method to generate a "personal" therapeutic tumor-specific vaccine. Two recent reports focused on this issue.

In one approach, in 2017 Patrick Ott and co-workers conducted whole-exome sequencing of DNA from matched tumor cells and normal cells from individuals to identify somatic mutations.[54] These potential tumor-specific neoantigens were then validated for actual expression by RNA sequencing of the tumor cells. To determine whether any of the expressed putative neoantigens would bind to HLA-A or B molecules of the individual, machine learning approaches were used. Clinical grade long peptides were synthesized with lengths of 15–30 amino acids, targeting up to 20 putative neoantigens, which were admixed with adjuvant poly-ICLC and grouped into four immunizing pools. Six subjects completed a series of five priming and two boosted vaccinations. After a median follow-up of 25 months, four subjects remained without disease recurrence. Two subjects had disease recurrence noted after restaging at the end of the vaccination interval, were treated with anti-PD-1 and achieved complete radiographic responses. Extensive *in vitro* testing by IFNγ ELISPOTs and intracellular cytokine staining detected by flow cytometry revealed that both CD4+ and CD8+ T cells were activated by the neoantigens in the vaccines. Thus, the investigators concluded that their study provided 'proof of principle' that a 'personal vaccine' can be produced and administered to individuals suffering from metastatic melanoma to generate highly specific immune responses against the individual's tumor.

In another approach reported in the same issue in 2017 by Ugur Sabin and colleagues, mutations expressed by 13 subjects with stage III and IV melanoma were identified by comparative exome and RNA sequencing of routine tumor biopsies and healthy blood cells.[55] Mutations were ranked according to predicted high affinity binding to autologous HLA Class I & II molecules. To create vaccines, ten selected mutations/subject were engineered into two synthetic RNAs, each encoding five linker-connected 27mer peptides with the mutation in position 14. At least eight doses of the neo-epitope vaccine were injected percutaneously into inguinal lymph nodes under ultrasound guidance. The immunogenicity of each of the mutations administered was analyzed by IFNγ ELISPOTs in CD4+ and CD8+ T cells in pre- and post-vaccination blood samples. Responses were detected against 60% of the predicted neo-epitopes, and each subject developed responses against at least three mutations. Eight subjects had no radiologically detectable lesions at start of vaccination and remained recurrence-free for the whole follow-up period (12–23 months). These investigators concluded that their study demonstrated the clinical feasibility and safety of targeting individual cancer mutations by RNA neo-epitope vaccines, thereby supporting the case for making individually-tailored medicines available to a wider range of patients.

References

1. Coley W. (1893). The treatment of malignant tumors by repeated inoculations of erysipalas: With a report of ten original cases. *Am J Med Sci* **10**:487–511.
2. Portier P and Richet C. (1902). De l'action anaphylactique de certains venims. *Comptes Rendus Soc Biol* **54**:170–172.
3. von Pirquet C and Shick B. (1951). *Serum Sickness*. Baltimore: The Williams and Wilkins Co.
4. Calmette A, Guerin C, Weill-Halle B, *et al*. (1924). Essais d'immunisation contre l'infection tuberculeuse. *Bulliten de l'Academie de Medicine* **91**:787–796.
5. Mathe G, Amiel J, Schwarzenberg L, *et al*. (1969). Active immunotherapy for acute lymphoblastic anemia. *The Lancet* **293**:697–699.
6. Rous P. (1911). A sarcoma of the fowl transmisable by an agent separable from the tumor cells. *J Exp Med* **132**:397–411.
7. Gillis S and Smith K. (1977). *In vitro* generation of tumor-specific cytotoxic lymphocytes. Secondary allogeneic mixed tumor lymphocyte culture of normal murine spleen cells. *J Exp Med* **146**:468–482.
8. Gillis S, Ferm MM, Ou W, and Smith KA. (1978). T cell growth factor: Parameters of production and a quantitative microassay for activity. *J Immunol* **120**:2027–2032.
9. Gillis S and Smith KA. (1977). Long term culture of tumour-specific cytotoxic T cells. *Nature* **268**:154–156.
10. Baker PE, Gillis S, and Smith, KA. (1979). Monoclonal cytolytic T-cell lines. *J Exp Med* **149**:273–278.
11. Billingham R, Silvers W, and Wilson D. (1962). Adoptive transfer of transplantation immunity by means of blood-borne cells. *The Lancet* **1**:512–515.
12. Robb RJ and Smith KA. (1981). Heterogeneity of human T-cell growth factor(s) due to variable glycosylation. *Mol Immunol* **18**:1087–1094.
13. Smith KA, Favata MF, and Oroszlan S. (1983). Production and characterization of monoclonal antibodies to human interleukin 2: Strategy and tactics. *J Immunol* **131**:1808–1815.

14. Robb RJ, Munck A, and Smith KA. (1981). T cell growth factor receptors: Quantitation, specificity, and biological relevance. *J Exp Med* **154**:1455–1474.

15. Taniguchi T, Matsui H, Fujita T, et al. (1983). Structure and expression of a cloned cDNA for human interleukin-2. *Nature* **302**:305–310.

16. Rosenberg SA, Lotze MT, Muul LM, et al. (1985). Observations on the systemic administration of autologous lymphokine-activated killer cells and recombinant interleukin-2 to patients with metastatic cancer. *N Engl J Med* **313**:1485–1492.

17. Caligiuri MA, Zmuidzinas A, Manley TJ, et al. (1990). Functional consequences of interleukin 2 receptor expression on resting human lymphocytes. Identification of a novel natural killer cell subset with high affinity receptors. *J Exp Med* **171**:1509–1526.

18. Zhang X, Sun S, Hwang I, et al. (1998). Potent and selective stimulation of memory-phenotype CD8+ T cells *in vivo* by IL-15. *Immunity* **8**:591–599.

19. Rosenberg SA, Lotze MT, Muul LM, et al. (1987). A progress report on the treatment of 157 patients with advanced cancer using lymphokine-activated killer cells and interleukin-2 or high-dose interleukin-2 alone. *N Engl J Med* **316**:889–897.

20. Klein E, Svedmyr E, Mikael J, and Vanky F. (1977). Functional studies on tumor infiltrating lymphocytes in man. *Israel J Med Sci* **13**:747–752.

21. Holmes E. (1985). Immunology of tumor infiltrating lymphocytes. *Cancer Res* **201**:158–163.

22. Miesher S, Whiteside T, Carrel S, and von Fliedner V. (1986). Functional properties of tumor-infiltrating and blood lymphocytes in patients with solid tumors: Effects of tumor cells and their supernatants on proliferative responses of lymphocytes. *J Immunol* **136**:1899–1907.

23. Rosenberg S, Spiess P, and Lafreniere R. (1986). A new approach to the adoptive immunotherapy of cancer with tumor-infiltrating lymphocytes. *Science* **233**:1318–1321.

24. Rosenberg S, Packard B, Aebersold P, et al. (1988). Use of tumor-infiltrating lymphocytes and interleukin-2 in the immunotherapy of patients with metastatic melanoma. *N Eng J Med* **319**:1676–1680.

25. Rosenberg S, Lotze M, Yang J, et al. (1989). Experience with the use of high dose interleukin-2 in the treatment of 652 cancer patients. *Ann Surg* **210**:474–485.

26. Rosenberg S, Lotze M, Yang J, et al. (1993). Prospective randomized trial of high dose interleukin-2 alone or in conjunction with lymphokine-activated killer cells for the treatment of patients with advanced cancer. *J Natl Cancer Inst* **85**:622–632.

27. Rooney C, Smith C, Ng, C, *et al.* (1995). Use of gene-modified virus-specific T lymphocytes to control Epstein-Barr-virus-related lymphoproliferation. *Lancet* **345**:9–13.

28. Walter E, Greenberg P, Gilbert M, *et al.* (1995). Reconstitution of cellular immunity against cytomegalovirus in recipients of allogeneic bone marrow by transfer of T-cell clones from the donor. *N Engl J Med* **333**:1038–1044.

29. Eshhar Z, Waks T, Gross G, and Schindler D. (1993). Specific activation and targeting of cytotoxic lymphocytes through chimeric single chains consisting of antibody-binding domains and the gamma or zeta subunits of the immunoglobulin and T-cell receptors. *Proc Natl Acad Sci USA* **90**:720–724.

30. Bejcek B, Wang D, Berven E, *et al.* (1995). Development and characterization of three recombinant single chain antibody fragments (scFvs) directed against the CD19 antigen. *Cancer Res* **55**:2346–2351.

31. Brentjens R, Latouche J-B, Santos E, *et al.* (2003). Eradication of systemic B-cell tumors by genetically targeted human T lymphocytes co-stimulated by CD80 and interleukin-15. *Nat Med* **9**:279–286.

32. Kohn D, Dotti G, Brentjens R, *et al.* (2011). CARs on track in the clinic. *Molec Ther* **19**:432–438.

33. Hu Y, Sun J, Wu Z, *et al.* 2016. Predominant cerebral cytokine release syndrome in CD19-directed chimeric antigen receptor-modified therapy. *J Hem & Onc* **9**:70.

34. Sommermyer D, Hill T, Shamah S, *et al.* (2017). Fully human CD19-specific chimeric antigen receptors for T cell therapy. *Leukemia* **1**:9.

35. Hanson H, Donermeyer D, Ikeda H, *et al.* (2000). Eradication of established tumors by CD8+ T cell adoptive immunotherapy. *Immunity* **13**:265–276.

36. Ikeda H, Ohta N, Furukawa K, *et al.* (1997). Mutated mitogen-activated protein kinase: A tumor rejection antigen of mouse sarcoma. *Proc Natl Acad Sci USA* **94**:6375–6379.

37. Kessels H, Wolkers M, van den Boom M, *et al.* (2001). Immunotherapy through TCR gene transfer. *Nat Immunol* **2**:957–961.

38. Ahmadzadeh M, Johnson L, Heemskerk B, *et al.* (2009). Tumor antigen-specific CD8+ T cells infiltrating the tumor express high levels of PD-1 and are functionally impaired. *Blood* **114**:1537–1544.

39. West E, Jin H-T, Rasheed A-U, *et al.* (2013). PD-L1 blockade synergizes with IL-2 therapy in invigorating exhausted T cells. *J Clin Invest.*

40. June C, Riddell S, and Schumacher T. (2015). Adoptive cellular therapy: A race to the finish line. *Sci Trans Med* **7**:280–287.

41. Phan GQ, Yang JC, Sherry RM, *et al.* (2003). Cancer regression and autoimmunity induced by cytotoxic T lymphocyte-associated antigen 4 blockade in patients with metastatic melanoma. *Proc Natl Acad Sci USA* **100**:8372–8377.

42. Tivol E, Borriello F, Schweitzer A, *et al.* (1995). Loss of CTLA-4 leads to massive lymphoproliferation and fatal multiorgan tissue destruction, revealing c critical negative regulatory role of CTLA-4. *Immunity* **3**:541–547.

43. Waterhouse P, Penningger J, Timms E, *et al.* (1995). Lymphoproliferative disorders with early lethality in mice deficient in CTLA-4. *Science* **270**:985–988.

44. Klocke K, Sakaguchi S, Holmdahl R, and Wing K. (2016). Induction of autoimmune disease by deletion of CTLA-4 in mice in adulthood. *Proc Natl Acad Sci USA* **113**:E2382–2392.

45. Hodi F, O'Day S, McDermott D, *et al.* (2010). Improved survival with ipiliumab in patients with metastatic melanoma. *N Eng J Med* **363**.

46. Voskens C, Goldinger S, Loquai C, *et al.* (2013). The price of tumor control: An analysis of rare side effects of anti-CTLA-4 therapy in metastatic melanoma. *PLOS ONE* **8**:e53745.

47. Schadendorf D, Hodi S, Robert C, *et al.* (2015). Pooled analysis of long-term survival data from phase II and phase III trials of ipimumab in unresectable or metastatic melanoma. *J Clin Onc* **33**:1889–1835.

48. Topalian S, Hodi F, Brahmer J, *et al.* (2012). Safety, activity, and immune correlates of anti-PD-1 antibody in cancer. *N Eng J Med* **366**:2443–2454.

49. Brahmer J, Tykodi S, Chow L, *et al.* (2012). Safety and activity of anti-PDL-1 antibody in patients with advanced cancer. *N Eng J Med* **366**:2455–2465.

50. Larkin J, Chiarion-Sileni R, Grob J, *et al.* (2015). Combined nivolmab and ipilimumab or monotherapy in untreated melanoma. *N Eng J Med* **373**:23–34.

51. Johnson D, Balko J, Compton M, *et al.* (2016). Fulminant myocarditis with combination immune checkpoint blockade. *N Eng J Med* **375**:1749–1755.

52. Rizvi N, Hellmann M, Snyder A, *et al.* (2015). Mutational landscape determines sensitivity to PD-1 blockade in non-small cell lung cancer. *Science* **348**:124–128.

53. Le D, Durham J, Smith K, *et al.* (2017). Mismatch-repair deficiency predicts response of solid tumors to PD-1 blockade. *Science* **357**:409–413.

54. Ott P, Hu Z, Keskin D, *et al*. (2017). An immunogenic personal neoantigen vaccine for patients with melanoma. *Nature* **547**:217–221.
55. Sahin U, Derhovanessian E, Miller M, *et al*. (2017). Personalized RNA mutanome vaccines mobilize poly-specific therapeutic immunity against cancer. *Nature* **547**:222–226.

Epilogue

For the past 60 years, immunology has been doing the work of Linnaeus, identifying, characterizing and cataloguing the cells and the molecules that make up the immune system. Now, the work of Darwin begins to discern how the total system is regulated. This more exciting new work is only possible now, because we have done the work of Linnaeus. Because of the capacity to delete individual genes in both embryos as well as fully grown animals, we have begun to appreciate the complexity of the immune system, as well as to anticipate the effects of suppressing or enhancing the function of some of the molecules we have discovered to design new immunotherapies for the first time. Again, this leap into therapy is only possible now that the work of Linnaeus has been accomplished taking immunology to the molecular, i.e. nm, level. For example, pharmacologic approaches to suppress both the production and action of cytokines have become standard to block organ transplant rejection, while other new agents have become useful to block cytokines or their receptors for the suppression of autoinflammatory and allergic diseases. Perhaps the most promising therapeutic manipulations of the immune system are new ways that have been discovered to augment immunoreactivity, so that the immune system can be harnessed to hopefully cure some patients suffering from cancer. At this stage, the field is in its infancy, but it is already clear that only a fraction of patients is helped by non-specifically augmenting immune recognition and responsivity by administering immune-enhancing cytokines or blocking negative feedback pathways. Most evidence indicates that those who are helped are those whose cancer cells have multiple mutations, so that mutant peptides are presented to the immune system on the cell surface, thereby capable of arousing T cell-mediated immunity. Accordingly, future work focused on identifying immunogenic mutant peptides that can be used as neoantigens for therapeutic vaccines may well create the therapies that can help most individuals suffering from cancer rather than just a minority. However, it seems clear that we must devise methods to activate a polyclonal immune response to cancer, so that we must identify multiple mutant neoantigens. Otherwise, the immunologically directed Darwinian selection of resistant cancer cell mutants will thwart our hopes for truly curative cancer immunotherapy. But, the future looks bright, in that there do not seem to be any remaining technological hurdles that must be surmounted. Moreover, the work of Darwin promises to be fun as well as fruitful for medicine.

Name Index

Subject Index

Printed in the United States
By Bookmasters